Diabetes

an

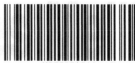

Incredibly Easy!™

MiniGuide

Springhouse Corporation
Springhouse, Pennsylvania

Staff

Vice President
Matthew Cahill

Clinical Director
Judith A. Schilling McCann,
RN, MSN

Art Director
John Hubbard

Executive Editor
Michael Shaw

Managing Editor
Andrew T. McPhee, RN,
BSN

Clinical Editors
Pamela Mullen Kovach, RN,
BSN; Carla M. Roy, RN,
BSN, CCRN

Editors
Craig Mongeau, Ed
Pratowski, Patricia Wittig

Copy Editors
Brenna H. Mayer (manager),
Gretchen Fee, Priscilla H.
Dewitt, Stacey A. Follin,
Pamela Wingrod

Designers
Arlene Putterman (associ-
ate art director), Mary
Ludwicki (book designer),
Joseph Clark, Jacalyn B.
Facciolo, Donna S. Morris

Illustrator,
Bot Roda, Betty Winnberg

Typography
Diane Paluba (manager),
Joyce Rossi Biletz, Valerie
Molettiere

Manufacturing
Deborah Meiris (director),
Patricia K. Dorshaw
(manager), Otto Mezei (book
production manager)

Editorial Assistants
Beverly Lane, Marcia Mills,
Liz Schaeffer

Indexer
Ellen Murray

for brief quotations embodied in
critical articles and reviews. For
information, write Springhouse
Corporation, 1111 Bethlehem Pike,
P.O. Box 908, Springhouse, PA
19477-0908. Authorization to photocopy items for internal or personal
use, or for the internal or personal
use of specific clients, is granted
by Springhouse Corporation for
users registered with the Copyright
Clearance Center (CCC)
Transactional Reporting Service,
provided that the fee of $.75 per
page is paid directly to CCC, 222
Rosewood Dr., Danvers, MA, 01923.
For those organizations that have
been granted a photocopy license
by CCC, a separate system of pay-
ment has been arranged. The fee
code for users of the Transactional
Reporting Service is 1-58255-012-
3/2000 $00.00 + .75.

Printed in the United States of
America.

IEMDM-010899

℞ A member of the Reed Elsevier plc group

**Library of Congress Cataloging-in
Publication Data**

Diabetes mellitus: an incredibly easy
miniguide
    p.   cm. — (Miniguides)
    Includes index.
    1. Diabetes Handbooks, manuals,
etc. I. Springhouse Corporation.
II. Series: Incredibly easy miniguide.
    [DNLM: 1. Diabetes Mellitus
    Handbooks. WK 39 D5355 1999]
RC660.M4546 1999
616.4'62—dc21
DNLM/DLC   99-27035
ISBN 1-58255-012-3 (alk. paper) CIP

Contents

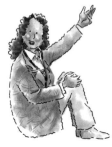

Contributors and Consultants

Joanne M. Bartelmo, RN, MSN, CCRN
Clinical Educator
Pottstown (Pa.) Memorial
Medical Center

Nancy Cirone, RN,C, MSN, CDE
Director of Education
Warminster (Pa.) Hospital

Margaret Friant Cramer, RN, MSN
Clinical Supervisor
Cardiac Solutions, Inc.
Fort Washington, Pa.

Michael Carter, RN, DNSc, FAAN
Dean and Professor
College of Nursing
University of Tennessee
Memphis

Pamela Mullen Kovach, RN, BSN
Independent Clinical
Consultant
Perkiomenville, Pa.

Patricia A. Lange, RN, MSN, EdD (candidate), **CS, CCRN**
Graduate Nursing Program
Coordinator and Assistant
Professor of Nursing
Hawaii Pacific University
Kaneohe

Mary Ann Siciliano McLaughlin, RN, MSN
Clinical Supervisor
Cardiac Solutions, Inc.
Fort Washington, Pa.

Lori Musolf Neri, RN, MSN, CCRN
Clinical Instructor
Villanova (Pa.) University

Joseph L. Neri, DO, FACC
Cardiologist
The Heart Care Group
Allentown, Pa.

Robert Rauch
Manager of Government
Economics
Amgen, Inc.
Thousand Oaks, Calif.

Larry E. Simmons, RN, PhD
(candidate)
Clinical Instructor
University of Missouri-
Kansas City

Foreword

Diabetes is the leading cause of adult blindness and end-stage renal disease in the United States. More than 15 million people in this country have diabetes but only two-thirds of them know it.

Meeting the challenges of caring for a patient with diabetes requires a full understanding of the disorder and its implications for care. At once accurate, authoritative, and completely up-to-date, *Diabetes Mellitus: An Incredibly Easy MiniGuide* can help you gain an in-depth understanding of diabetes in an amazingly fun and exciting way.

The first chapter, *Understanding diabetes,* lays the foundation for your understanding by providing basic facts about the pathophysiology of diabetes and the effects of diabetes on the body. The next three chapters cover prevention, assessment, and treatment of diabetes. The fifth chapter covers complications of the disorder, and the final chapter covers patient teaching.

Throughout the book, you'll find features designed to make learning about diabetes lively and entertaining. For instance, *Memory joggers* provide clever tricks for remembering key points. Checklists, rendered in the style of a classroom chalkboard, provide at-a-glance summaries of important facts.

Cartoon characters that nearly pop off the page provide light-hearted chuckles as well as reinforcement of essential material. And a *Quick quiz* at the end of every chapter gives you a chance to assess your learning and refresh your memory at the same time.

The depth of information contained in this truly pocket-sized guide will impress even the most experienced health care professional. If you want a quick-learn, comprehensive reference about one of the most common conditions encountered in health care, I can't think of a more fitting resource than *Diabetes Mellitus: An Incredibly Easy MiniGuide.* It packs a wallop.

Michael Carter, RN, DNSc, FAAN
Dean and Professor
College of Nursing
University of Tennessee
Memphis

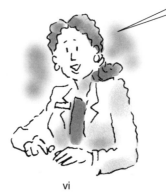

Professional development that's fun and exciting? Incredible!

Understanding diabetes

Key facts
♦ Diabetes mellitus occurs when the body can't make use of glucose in the blood-stream.

♦ The most common forms of diabetes are type 1 (formerly known as insulin-dependent or juvenile-onset diabetes) and type 2 (formerly known as non-insulin-dependent or adult-onset diabetes).

♦ Insufficient insulin levels occur when beta cells in the pancreas fail to produce enough insulin or receptor sites are insensitive to insulin.

♦ Lack of proper glucose control can lead to a wide range of problems, including a danger-ous state called hyperosmolar hyperglyce-mic nonketotic syndrome.

What is diabetes?

The term *diabetes mellitus* refers to a group of diseases characterized by high blood glucose levels (hyperglycemia). (*Note:* Most mentions of the term *dia-*

betes refer to diabetes mellitus, not diabetes insipidus, a separate disorder not discussed in this book.) Diabetes is the leading cause of adult blindness and end-stage renal disease in the United States. Most people with diabetes — 90 % — have type 2 diabetes, which occurs during adulthood.

It's diabetes, dontcha know?

More than 15 million people have diabetes but only two-thirds of them know it. (See *Who has diabetes?*) The number of people who develop diabetes has been increasing by about 8% per year. That increase is due in part to a growing population of older people and an increasing number of obese individuals. Age and obesity play key roles in the development of diabetes.

Patients with diabetes typically seek treatment when they develop complications of the disease.

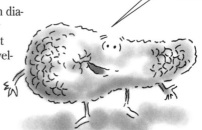

I cause a lot of problems in a lot of people, a bunch of whom don't even know it!

Who has diabetes?

Diabetes affects more than 15 million people in the United States. This chart outlines the number of people in selected high risk populations.

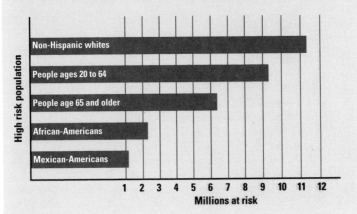

Types and causes of diabetes

Types of diabetes can be categorized by the pathology behind them and when they occur. The categories include:

👆 type 1 (insulin-dependent) diabetes

👆 type 2 (non-insulin-dependent) diabetes

gestational diabetes mellitus (GDM)

 secondary diabetes.

Type 1 diabetes

Type 1 diabetes, accounting for about 10% of diabetes cases, affects primarily young people, though it can arise at any age. This form of diabetes was formerly called juvenile diabetes, juvenile-onset diabetes, ketosis-prone diabetes, and unstable or brittle diabetes.

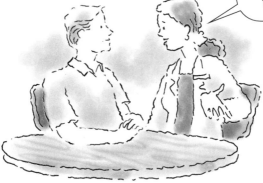

Characteristics of type 1

In type 1 diabetes, the onset of symptoms typically occurs without warning. Pancreatic beta cells, which normally produce insulin, become unable to produce insulin. As a result, the patient becomes dependent on exogenous insulin. Generally, beta cell destruction occurs at a faster rate in children than in adults.

So, why do I have type 1?

The cause of type 1 diabetes is unknown. The disorder has been associated with several genetic markers including human leukocyte antigens on chromosome 6, which contains genes that control the

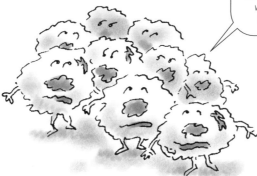

Please don't think we're giving up on you. We want to make insulin for you, but we just can't.

body's immune response. One theory suggests that circulating islet cell antibodies and anti-insulin antibodies apparently identify pancreatic cells as foreign bodies and then destroy them.

Type 1 diabetes may also develop as a result of infection or toxic environmental injury in a person genetically predisposed to develop an autoimmune response to beta cells. For instance, antibodies produced after a viral infection may attack beta cells and damage them enough to cause diabetes. The fact that immunosuppressive drugs slow the progression of diabetes supports this theory.

Type 2 diabetes

Type 2 diabetes has been called adult-onset diabetes, maturity-onset diabetes, ketosis-resistant diabetes, and stable diabetes. Type 2 diabetes is a milder form of diabetes that occurs mainly in adults but can also affect children.

Hmmm, am I destroying my own cells? Only time and further research will tell.

Now I get it!

Type 2 diabetes and obesity

Most patients with type 2 diabetes are obese. Because insulin resistance decreases with exercise and weight loss, researchers believe obesity promotes insulin resistance.

Obesity leads to increased levels of circulating insulin, primarily due to insulin being secreted in response to carbohydrate ingestion. High levels of insulin cause a decrease in the number of insulin receptor sites available, which in turn leads to insulin resistance and resultant hyperglycemia.

Type 2 diabetes and the nonobese patient

The exact cause of nonobese type 2 diabetes is largely unknown. Several rare genetic abnormalities have been discovered among nonobese type 2 diabetic patients. These abnormalities may play a role in the development of the disease in these individuals.

Characteristics of type 2

In type 2 diabetes, onset of the disease is gradual and typically causes vague signs and symptoms. Insufficient insulin activity exists to meet the body's demands.

Type 2 diabetes occurs mainly in obese individuals over age 40 who have a strong family history of the disease. (See *Type 2 diabetes and obesity.*) The disease can also affect nonobese individuals of any age. Most newly diagnosed patients have had the disease for a decade or more and are already experiencing long-term vascular and neuropathic complications by the time a diagnosis is made.

Tell me again. What causes this?

Doctors aren't sure what the exact cause of type 2 diabetes is, but common to type 1 and type 2 is a tissue insensitivity to insulin, called insulin resistance. This may be the result of a genetic factor aggravated over time by other factors, such as aging and obesity.

Another theory

Researchers are also looking into the existence of beta cell defects or peripheral site defects. Defects in beta cells would alter insulin secretion and change the quantity or quality of insulin produced. Defects at peripheral sites would limit insulin's ability to bind to cell walls.

Syndrome X files

High levels of circulating insulin and glucose indicate impaired glucose tolerance (IGT) and are thought to predispose a patient to syndrome X. This syndrome consists of a combination of disorders — IGT, high blood pressure, dyslipidemia, and central obesity — that puts the patient at a high risk for cardiac problems. Keep in mind that macrovascular complications arising from these disorders accounts for 75% of deaths from diabetes.

GDM

GDM occurs during pregnancy and usually disappears following delivery. Many women diagnosed with GDM develop diabetes later in life. Symptoms are usually mild, though untreated GDM can cause a number of complications. For instance, even mildly elevated glucose levels are associated with increased fetal morbidity.

Secondary diabetes

Diabetes can arise as a secondary condition as well — after a bout with an unrelated disease or condition or as a result of certain treatments. For instance, secondary diabetes can arise from pancreatic disease or hormonal or genetic syndromes, or from the ingestion of drugs, such as corticosteroids and thiazide diuretics. In most cases, secondary diabetes disappears when the underlying condition is corrected.

Causes

Causes of secondary diabetes include:
- physical or emotional stress that may lead to prolonged elevated levels of stress hormones (cortisol, epinephrine, glucagon, and growth hormone)
- higher levels of the body's stress hormones that lead to elevations in blood glucose, thereby increasing demands on the pancreas
- certain medications (including thiazide diuretics, adrenal corticosteroids, and oral contraceptives) that antagonize the effects of insulin.

Pathophysiology

Diabetes is a progressive disease that follows the same course in every patient, regardless of the cause or type of diabetes. Insulin and glucose are the two key players in all forms of the condition.

Insulin ins and outs

Understanding diabetes requires an understanding of insulin. Here are some facts about this key hormone:

(Text continues on page 19.)

Pancreatic cells

he pancreas is made up of pancreatic acini (tissues that secrete digestive enzymes
to the duodenum) and islets of Langerhans (tissues that secrete insulin and glucagon
irectly into the bloodstream). Each islet consists of alpha, beta, and delta cells, each of
/hich has a different function. This illustration shows a single islet of Langerhans and
e various types of cells found in it.

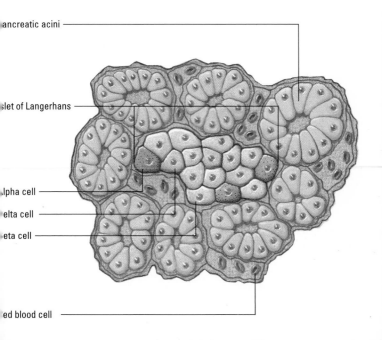

ancreatic acini

slet of Langerhans

lpha cell

elta cell

eta cell

ed blood cell

How antibodies attack islet cells

In type I diabetes, beta cells in the islets of Langerhans are attacked directly by the body's own antibodies, called autoantibodies. These autoantibodies bind to a substance inside the beta cell and destroy the cell. If enough cells are destroyed, the pancreas can no longer produce insulin. This illustration shows how an autoantibody attaches to a particular receptor on the beta cell membrane. Once attached, the autoantibody enters the cell and destroys it.

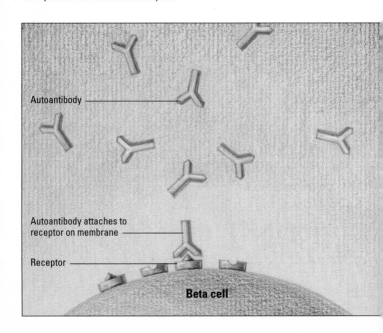

Autoantibody

Autoantibody attaches to receptor on membrane

Receptor

Beta cell

Insulin resistance

Insulin resistance is the major characteristic of type 2 diabetes. In insulin resistance, the amount of insulin produced by the pancreas may be normal, decreased, or even increased. However, the insulin is unable to bind with receptor sites. If the insulin can't bind with a receptor, glucose outside the cell can't pass through the cell membrane and be used by the cell for energy.

Insulin's inability to bind to receptor sites may be attributed to a defect at the receptor site, a decreased number of receptor sites, or a defect at the postreceptor site located inside the cell. These illustrations show the role of receptor sites in a normal cell and in insulin-resistant cells.

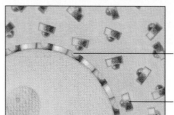

Normal

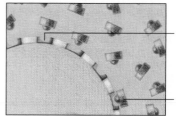

Defective receptors

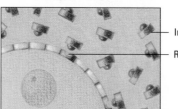

Too few receptors

Physiology of food ingestion

In a nondiabetic person, the ingestion of food triggers a predictable series of events, including the conversion of glucose into energy and the storage of glucose as glycogen. This illustration highlights this series of events.

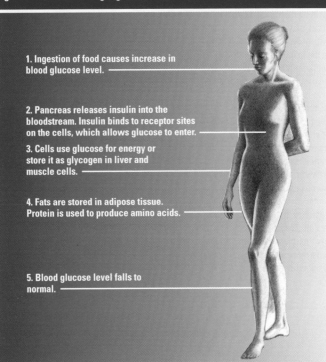

1. Ingestion of food causes increase in blood glucose level. ——————

2. Pancreas releases insulin into the bloodstream. Insulin binds to receptor sites on the cells, which allows glucose to enter. ——

3. Cells use glucose for energy or store it as glycogen in liver and muscle cells. ——————

4. Fats are stored in adipose tissue. Protein is used to produce amino acids. ——————

5. Blood glucose level falls to normal. ——————

Abnormal response to food ingestion

In a person with diabetes, the body's normal response to food ingestion is altered. This illustration shows the changes that occur in how the body handles the fats, proteins, and carbohydrates ingested as food.

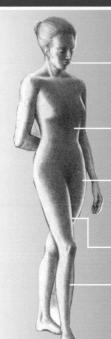

1. Ingestion of food causes increase in blood glucose level.

2. Little or no insulin is released or problems exist in insulin receptor sites. As a result, cells are unable to use or store glucose and the glucose level remains high.

3. Cells become starved for energy. Fats and proteins are used for energy rather than being stored.

4. Amino acids are broken down into glucose and other components. Free fatty acids released by adipose tissue are converted by the liver to ketone bodies, for use as energy.

5. Blood glucose level continues to rise.

How complications arise

Sustained high blood glucose levels can cause — in as little as 2 years after onset of the disease — a series of damaging effects at the cellular level. These effects accumulate and may eventually cause complications, including retinopathy and nephropathy. The illustrations below highlight the effects of sustained hyperglycemia on cells.

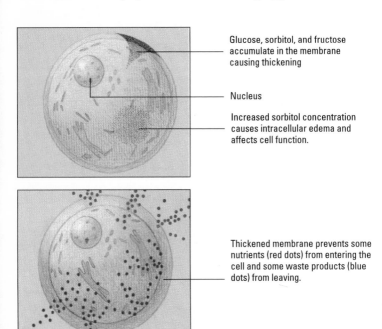

Glucose, sorbitol, and fructose accumulate in the membrane causing thickening

Nucleus

Increased sorbitol concentration causes intracellular edema and affects cell function.

Thickened membrane prevents some nutrients (red dots) from entering the cell and some waste products (blue dots) from leaving.

Systemic response to low blood glucose

The body of a person who doesn't have diabetes reacts to a low blood glucose level with a predictable series of events that starts when the brain senses a drop in the level of blood glucose. This illustration shows the normal response to hypoglycemia.

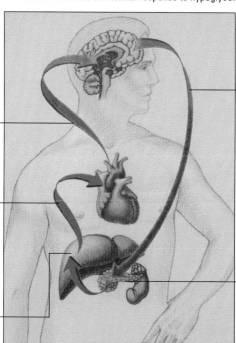

5. Increased blood glucose sensed by brain, which adjusts counter-measures accordingly.

1. Brain senses drop in blood glucose and signals pancreas to react.

4. Blood glucose level increases.

2. Alpha cells in the pancreas release glucagon into bloodstream.

3. Glucagon prompts liver to break down glycogen into glucose.

Systemic response to low blood glucose *(continued)*

This illustration shows the response of a person with type 1 diabetes to hypoglycemia.

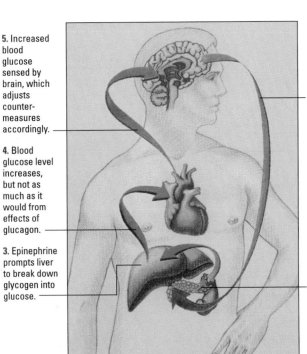

5. Increased blood glucose sensed by brain, which adjusts countermeasures accordingly.

1. Brain senses drop in blood glucose and signals pancreas to react.

4. Blood glucose level increases, but not as much as it would from effects of glucagon.

2. Pancreas fails to release glucagon. As a result, adrenal glands release epinephrine into bloodstream.

3. Epinephrine prompts liver to break down glycogen into glucose.

- Insulin is a hormone produced in areas of specialized tissue called islets of Langerhans, located throughout the pancreas.
- Beta cells in the islets of Langerhans produce insulin. Alpha cells produce glucagon, a hormone that increases the circulating levels of blood glucose.
- Insulin secretion rises in response to food.
- An increase in insulin levels causes a resulting decrease in blood glucose levels as glucose is transported into cells and used for energy. (See *How glucose enters cells,* page 20.)
- As blood glucose levels decrease, insulin levels decrease.

Let's take a look at the roles insulin and glucose play in the body.

More on insulin

Among its many other functions, insulin also:

- promotes the entry of amino acids into cells
- inhibits the destruction of proteins
- decreases the rate at which amino acids are released from cells
- inhibits the rate at which glucose is produced by the liver

Warning!

How glucose enters cells

Glucose is normally transported into cells when the cells need energy. Areas on the outer part of the cell that allow the cell to bind with insulin are called insulin receptors. When the cell and insulin bind together, glucose can enter the cell.

No insulin, no entry

Without insulin, glucose can't enter a cell. As a result, the glucose remains trapped in the blood. Some eventually spills into the urine as the kidneys try to flush out the extra glucose.

• promotes the conversion of glucose into fatty acids (a process called lipogenesis).

Gettin' down with glucose

Here are some key points about glucose, the body's main source of energy.

• Glucose is the body's main source of energy.

• Excess glucose is stored in the liver, with the assistance of insulin.

• Glucose in the liver is converted into glycogen (the storage form of

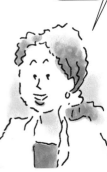

When glucose levels go up, insulin levels should go up. When glucose levels go down, insulin levels go down.

glucose) in a process called glycogenesis.

• When glucose levels fall, the liver converts glycogen back into glucose through the process of glycogenolysis. (See *Glycogen breakdown*, page 22.)

> Diabetes can occur if I don't produce enough insulin or the right quality of insulin.

Insufficient insulin action

A condition of insufficient insulin action occurs when beta cells fail to produce the right amount or quality of insulin. Insufficient insulin also occurs as a result of peripheral cell insulin resistance. Either way, insufficient amounts of insulin alter carbohydrate, protein, and fat metabolism.

Memory jogger

To remember the normal relationship of glucose and insulin, think of when Siskel and Ebert both loved a movie or both hated it. They gave it "two thumbs up" (glucose up, insulin up) or "two thumbs down" (insulin down, glucose down).

Now I get it!

Glycogen breakdown

The body can't differentiate between a glucose shortage and unusable insulin. In response to signs that the cells are starving, the liver converts stored glycogen to glucose, to increase the amount of glucose available to cells. Hyperglycemia then worsens because more glucose enters the bloodstream.

Starving cells

Glucose-starved cells lack the energy to function. The body attempts to compensate for this deficit by breaking down protein. Proteins are used by the cell for growth and repair of damages. Protein breakdown allows the liver to form new glucose molecules from amino acids.

Fats as an alternative fuel

Unlike protein, fats can be used by most cells as a direct source of energy. However, fats aren't efficient as a cellular fuel. They break down into free fatty acids and glycerol, a glucose-like substance that exacerbates hyperglycemia.

The further breakdown of free fatty acids produces ketone bodies, a waste product. The buildup of ketones causes the blood to become increasingly acidic.

Effects of cell starvation

When the blood glucose level rises, a predictable series of events occurs. (See *How hormones react to cell starvation,* page 25.)

Feeeeed me glucose! Without it, I have no energy and have to use protein for fuel. Ptoooie!

An increased blood glucose level causes osmotic diuresis, in which fluid is drawn from intracellular and interstitial spaces into the intravascular space.

Osmotic pressure in the extracellular fluid increases and, as it does, water moves out of the cells.

An increase in the amount of glucose passing through the renal tubules blocks fluid reabsorption there, causing diuresis.

Making matters worse

A number of counterregulatory hormones kick into action as a result of cell starvation and end up sustaining the hyperglycemia. Glucagon, epinephrine, cortisol and, to a lesser extent, growth hormone all oppose the action of insulin.

The cycle continues

Continued hyperglycemia and osmotic diuresis set up a relentless cycle of events interrupted only when the patient receives insulin. The massive fluid loss from osmotic diuresis causes fluid and electrolyte imbalances and dehydration, which further decreases renal excretion of glucose.

Water loss exceeds glucose and electrolyte loss, contributing to hyperosmolarity. This, in turn, worsens dehydration, decreasing the glomerular filtration rate and reducing the amount of glucose excreted in the urine.

Diminished glucose excretion further raises blood glucose levels, producing hyperosmolarity and dehydration and, if not treated, finally causing shock, coma, and death.

How hormones react to cell starvation

A variety of hormones affects glucose production and function. This chart lists the hormones and describes their effects on blood glucose.

Hormone	Effect
Glucagon	• Increases blood glucose concentration by causing glycogenolysis and increasing gluconeogenesis.
Epinephrine	• Stimulates glucagon release. • Inhibits insulin release.
Cortisol	• Stimulates glucagon release. • Decreases glucose utilization by the cells.
Somatostatin	• Inhibits the release of growth hormone from the anterior pituitary gland; also inhibits the release of certain hormones, such as glucagon and insulin.

Compensatory mechanisms

Ketosis results in metabolic acidosis with excess hydrogen ion concentration. The kidneys try to compensate for the acidosis by getting rid of ketones and ammonia. The lungs also compensate by getting rid of carbon dioxide (which promotes acidosis) through rapid, deep

Now I get it!

How diabetic ketoacidosis occurs

In type 1 diabetes, fat breakdown occurs so quickly that the liver can't handle the excess ketone bodies. Ketone bodies then spill into the bloodstream, causing ketoacidosis. Significant hyperglycemia in the presence of ketonemia is known as diabetic ketoacidosis.

In type 2 diabetes, the limited ability of the cells to use insulin allows the cells to function, if only sluggishly. Ketoacidosis usually doesn't occur in patients with type 2 diabetes unless they develop sepsis or experience extreme stress.

respirations, called Kussmaul's respirations.

When hyperglycemia progresses

As hyperglycemia progresses to diabetic ketoacidosis, the cardiac output decreases as a result of volume depletion. (See *How diabetic ketoacidosis occurs*.) Reduced cardiac output produces hypotension and reduced vital organ perfusion. Mental changes occur and may range from confusion to coma. If

As my output decreases, hypotension sets in and diminishes vital organ perfusion.

the condition remains untreated, death results.

Hyperosmolar hyperglycemic nonketotic syndrome

Hyperosmolar hyperglycemic nonketotic syndrome (HHNS), also known as hyperosmolar coma or hyperosmolar nonketotic syndrome, involves the development of severe hyperglycemia without ketonemia. (See *Hyperglycemic emergency,* page 28.) The reasons for this are unclear.

Who gets HHNS?

HHNS typically occurs in middle-aged or elderly patients. It may be the first appearance of diabetes in the patient or a severe exacerbation of previously mild, non-insulin-dependent diabetes.

HHNS can also occur in anyone whose insulin tolerance is stressed (as can happen in illness or trauma) and in patients who have undergone certain therapeutic procedures, such as peritoneal dialysis, hemodialysis, tube feedings, and total parenteral nutrition.

HHNS may be the first sign of diabetes in a patient.

Warning!

Hyperglycemic emergency

Hyperosmolar hyperglycemic nonketotic syndrome (HHNS) is an emergency condition that causes impaired consciousness.

Glycosuria tends to be worse in HHNS than in diabetic ketoacidosis because blood glucose levels are higher in HHNS. The clinical effects of HHNS result from:

- hyperosmolarity
- severe hyperglycemia
- severe dehydration from osmotic diuresis.

Quick quiz

1. In the United States, most people with diabetes have a form known as:

    A.   type 1 diabetes.

    B.   type 2 diabetes.

    C.   gestational diabetes mellitus.

Answer: B. About 90% of people with diabetes have type 2 (non-insulin-dependent) diabetes.

2. The main condition common to both type 1 diabetes and type 2 diabetes involves:
- A. inability of the pancreas to produce insulin.
- B. insensitivity of cells to the effects of insulin.
- C. ineffectiveness of insulin produced by the pancreas.

Answer: B. Common to type 1 and type 2 diabetes is a tissue insensitivity to insulin, called insulin resistance. This may be the result of a genetic factor aggravated over time by other factors, such as aging and obesity.

3. Polyuria, dehydration, and electrolyte imbalances in a person with diabetes occur as a result of:
- A. bicarbonate excretion.
- B. ketoacidosis.
- C. osmotic diuresis.

Answer: C. Osmotic diuresis occurs during hyperglycemia, causing polyuria, dehydration, and electrolyte imbalances. If the hyperglycemia continues, cardiac output decreases and hypotension and circulatory collapse can occur.

Scoring

☆☆☆ If you answered all three questions correctly, hip hip hooray! You've just been named Dean of the Institute of Osmotic Diuresis at DM University! Wow!

☆☆ If you answered two questions correctly, take a bow. You're the newest faculty member of the HHNS Center for Counterregulatory Hormones. Cool.

☆ If you answered fewer than two questions correctly, don't despair. We've got our eye on you as a visiting professor for the National Islets of Langerhans. We think you'll like it there.

2

Preventing diabetes

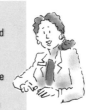

Key facts
- ◆ Early identification, prompt treatment, and early and consistent glucose control can prevent long-term complications.
- ◆ Chronic complications of diabetes include blindness, myocardial infarction, stroke, end-stage renal disease, nervous system abnormalities, and limb amputation.
- ◆ Even when a patient complies completely with treatment regimens, complications and death can result.

Understanding diabetes prevention

Diabetes prevention can be interpreted as preventing the disease, delaying its onset, or preventing or delaying the onset of complications. Prevention of diabetes is difficult. Several studies have shown that regular physical activity can significantly reduce the risk of developing type 2 diabetes. Weight reduction in obese individuals also appears to reduce that risk.

Currently, national studies are underway to determine whether type 1 or type 2 diabetes can be prevented.

Identifying risk factors

The primary preventive measure for individuals who may develop diabetes is to identify risk factors. (See *Screening high-risk children*.) Groups at high risk for developing diabetes include:
- Blacks, Hispanics, and Native Americans
- obese individuals

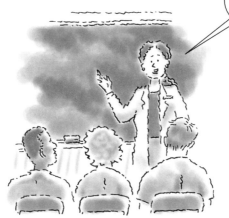

People at high risk for developing diabetes include blacks, obese individuals, and women who've given birth to large babies.

Advice from the experts

Screening high-risk children

The preferred method for screening high-risk children for diabetes involves testing them for the presence of islet cell antibodies. A positive test means that antibodies have already begun attacking the insulin-producing beta cells. Keep these points in mind when screening children for diabetes:

• An asymptomatic child doesn't need to be screened for type 1 diabetes, even if he has a family history of the disease.
• Siblings of a known diabetic don't require routine screening.
• Blood glucose testing in children should be done as soon as signs or symptoms appear.

• individuals who have a close relative with diabetes
• individuals with high blood pressure (140/90 mm Hg or higher)
• individuals with high serum levels of high-density lipoprotein (HDL; 35 mg/dl or higher) or triglycerides (250 mg/dl or higher)
• individuals who had impaired glucose tolerance or impaired fasting glucose on previous tests
• women who delivered a baby weighing more than 9 lb (4.1 kg)

• women diagnosed with gestational diabetes mellitus (GDM).

Who should be screened?

Diabetes — especially type 2 — often causes no obvious signs or symptoms. Because undetected diabetes can have devastating consequences, laboratory screening is recommended for the following groups:

• adults over age 45 (if normal, repeat testing every 3 years)
• obese individuals
• patients with a family history of diabetes
• patients with impaired glucose tolerance
• members of high risk ethnic groups
• patients with a blood lipid abnormality
• women with a history of obstetric complications or GDM
• women who delivered a baby weighing over 9 lb (4.1 kg)
• pregnant women during the 24th to 28th week of gestation. (Earlier screening is necessary for pregnant women who develop signs and symptoms before

this time, or who have an increased risk for diabetes.)

Modifying risk factors

Some risk factors for diabetes can be modified, thus preventing the onset of disease or slowing the onset of complications. Modifying those risk factors involves controlling blood glucose levels, maintaining a healthy diet, controlling weight, staying active, managing stress, and reducing the risk of cardiovascular complications.

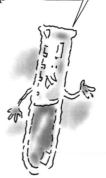

Using blood tests to screen for diabetes can help identify high-risk individuals.

Controlling glucose

Teach the patient at high risk for developing diabetes to monitor his blood glucose levels. Maintaining a normal blood glucose level reduces the risk of hyperglycemic episodes, which may place undue stress on the pancreas and promote earlier development of diabetes.

Insulin therapy *before diabetes sets in?*

Some high-risk patients, particularly those at risk for type 1 diabetes, may also benefit from insulin therapy before signs of diabetes appear. (See *Predicting type 1 diabetes.*) Insulin therapy for these patients helps relieve the pancreas of the burden of producing normal amounts of insulin and may prevent the onset of diabetes completely.

Healthy diet

A well-balanced diet also plays an important role in preventing complications of diabetes. For instance, choosing high-fiber foods instead of processed carbohydrates may dramatically reduce a woman's risk of developing type 2 diabetes. Fiber protects against diabetes by

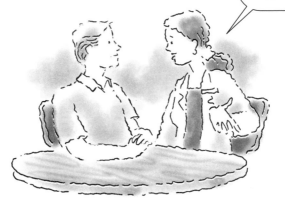

Now I get it!

Predicting type 1 diabetes

A protein molecule found on the surface of some white blood cells may reveal a person's risk of developing type 1 diabetes. If a person inherits one form of this protein molecule — HLA-DQ — he will be resistant to type 1 diabetes. If he inherits any of the other three forms of the molecule, however, he'll be more likely to develop the disease.

Study reveals key to diabetes risk

The chemical makeup of one region on the HLA-DQ molecule appears to hold the key, though scientists don't yet understand why. In one study, nondiabetic patients all possessed HLA-DQ molecules containing aspartic acid.

At least 90% of diabetics in the same study possessed HLA-DQ molecules containing one of three other amino acids: alanine, serine, or valine. Using highly sophisticated molecular techniques, researchers can accurately predict a person's susceptibility to type 1 diabetes.

slowing carbohydrate absorption, thus reducing demands on the pancreas.

Getting those fats in line

A low-cholesterol diet may be recommended to decrease low-density lipoprotein (LDL) levels to under 130 mg/dl and triglyceride levels to under 400 mg/dl, and increase HDL levels to above 35 mg/dl in men and above 45 mg/dl in women.

Reducing LDL and triglyceride levels and increasing HDL levels decreases the potential for developing cardiovascular problems and helps to stabilize blood glucose levels.

Exercise

Exercise decreases an individual's risk for developing type 2 diabetes as well as cardiovascular disease. Exercise effectively lowers blood glucose levels by enhancing glucose uptake in exercising muscles and increasing the body's sensitivity to insulin.

Exercising and controlling your weight are keys to preventing diabetes.

Richard Simmons would be proud!

Keep these important points in mind about exercise and diabetes:
• Exercise should be done regularly and consistently to enhance the effectiveness of the body's ability to reduce blood glucose levels and to avoid problems associated with glucose instability.
• Because exercise can result in hypoglycemia, the patient should check his blood glucose level before and after exercising.

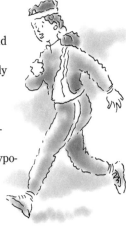

• Exercise can result in lowered blood glucose levels for up to 24 hours.
• Regular exercise may reduce the need for insulin.
• Exercise helps reduce blood glucose levels only when sufficient amounts of insulin are available. (In a patient with chronic hyperglycemia with a blood glucose level consistently above 300 mg/dl, exercise may lead to more severe hyperglycemia.)
• Aerobic exercise — such as walking, running, cycling, or swimming — is preferable because it uses glucose as fuel and helps lower blood glucose levels.

And that's not all

Other benefits of exercise include:
• decreased blood pressure
• weight reduction
• strengthening of the cardiovascular system, an important benefit because a patient with diabetes is at an increased risk for developing cardiovascular disease.

Weight reduction

A key predisposing factor in the development of type 2 diabetes is obesity. Of all patients with type 2 diabetes, 80% are obese. Obesity is a major cause of insulin resistance, so weight control plays a key role in controlling blood glucose levels. Weight reduction can also help reverse impaired glucose tolerance in obese diabetics.

Encourage your obese patient with type 2 diabetes to begin a weight reduction program. Supply information about such programs in the area, and follow the patient's progress.

Stress management

Stress increases blood glucose levels as a result of the demands it places on the entire body. Although the patient may not be able to control stress factors in his life, he can control the way he responds to stress through relaxation techniques and stress management.

Heart health

Controlling risk factors that contribute to cardiovascular disease may prove highly beneficial to the patient

Fighting stress with relaxation and stress-management techniques really does work.

with diabetes. Contributing risk factors include:

• dyslipidemia; contributes to the development of cardiovascular disease

• obesity; places an increased workload on the heart and vascular system

• sedentary lifestyle; increases the risk of developing heart disease

• smoking; alters peripheral circulation by constricting blood vessels and compromising cells distal to the constriction.

Preventing complications

To prevent or delay the onset of complications, teach the patient to understand the importance of carefully monitoring and controlling blood glucose levels. Three approaches are key to preventing long-term damage from complications of diabetes:

Improve maintenance of diabetes before complications develop.

Detect physical changes early on that point to complications.

Promptly treat complications.

Preventable problems?

Complications that maybe prevented or delayed in a patient with diabetes include:

- foot problems
- infection
- nephropathy
- neuropathy
- retinopathy.

Diabetic foot problems

A patient with a foot ulcer or history of a foot ulcer or pain in his calf or thigh

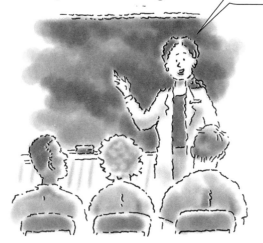

To prevent or delay complications, you need to monitor and control your blood glucose levels carefully.

when walking is in a high-risk category for progressive foot problems, possibly leading to amputation. Foot problems frequently encountered by patients with diabetes include:

- impaired circulation
- infection
- paresthesia
- reduced sensation
- ulcer.

Daily inspection of the feet is critical for detecting problems early.

So, how do my toes look today?

Because of the increased risk of foot problems, patients with diabetes should have a thorough examination of their feet regularly. Other preventive measures include:

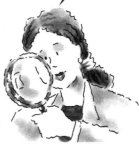

- daily washing of the feet, taking care to dry thoroughly between the toes
- daily inspection of the feet for corns, calluses, redness, swelling, bruises, and breaks in the skin
- reporting changes to the primary care provider
- never walking barefoot
- always wearing socks with shoes
- having a podiatrist remove corns and calluses

• cutting toenails straight across
• wearing comfortable, nonconstricting shoes. (Keep in mind that Medicare may pay for therapeutic shoes for patients with diabetes.)

Infection

Diabetic patients face a considerably higher risk of bacterial infection than nondiabetic patients do. (See *Infection and diabetes.*) When teaching patients about reducing risks of infection, be sure to cover these points:
• Provide meticulous skin and foot care.
• Keep the hands and feet warm in cold weather.
• Avoid the use of hot water bottles and heating pads to reduce the risk of burns stemming from reduced skin sensitivity.
• For female patients, avoid bubble baths and wear cotton undergarments to prevent vaginitis.
• Wash your hands frequently, especially if someone in the household is ill.
• If a break in the skin occurs, wash the area with warm water and soap, dry the area, and apply a dry, sterile dressing. Change the dressing several times a day. Notify the primary care provider if the

Now I get it!

Infection and diabetes

Infection may be more prevalent in patients with diabetes than nondiabetics for a number of reasons.

• When the integrity of the skin is compromised, tissue hypoxia increases the risk of skin structure infections. In addition, the presence of glycosylated hemoglobin in red blood cells impairs the release of oxygen to tissues.

• Increased amounts of glucose in body fluids promotes the growth of certain organisms. The organisms thrive on the glucose, which they use for energy.

• Impairments in vision and touch reduce the body's ability to detect or react to dangers in the environment. Breaks in the skin occur as a result and can set the stage for infection.

• White blood cells (WBCs) don't work as well as they should in people with diabetes. Diffusion through the cell membrane becomes more difficult, and the abilities of phagocytic WBCs are impaired.

• Vascular changes in patients with diabetes lead to reduced blood flow to affected areas, decreasing the number of WBCs available to fight infection.

area becomes reddened, hot, swollen, or painful, or if drainage is present.

Retinopathy

Controlling hypertension helps prevent diabetic retinopathy and the blindness that can result. (See *Insulin resistance and hypertension.*) In patients with diabetes, retinopathy may involve microaneurysms, intraretinal hemorrhages, and macular edema or neovascularization of the retina and optic disk, vitreous hemorrhage, and retinal detachment. Aggressive control of blood glucose in patients with type 2 diabetes significantly reduces the chance of developing diabetic retinopathy as well as kidney failure.

Teach patients to immediately report visual problems so that prompt treatment can be started to prevent further damage. In addition, explain the importance

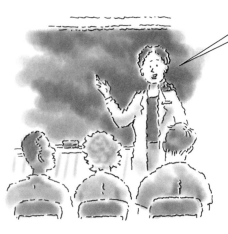

Infections pose a major threat to people with diabetes. You'll need to avoid infections as much as possible.

Battling illness

Insulin resistance and hypertension

Insulin resistance and the hyperinsulinemia that results may lead to hypertension in some patients with diabetes and some nondiabetic patients as well. Insulin resistance may contribute to hypertension by:

- promoting renal sodium retention
- altering vascular reactivity, which leads to constriction of renal arterioles
- stimulating catecholamine release.

Benefits of treatment

Controlling hypertension reduces the risk of:

- cardiovascular disease
- cerebrovascular disease
- diabetic nephropathy
- hypertensive nephropathy.

of regular eye examinations to detect early signs of retinopathy.

Nephropathy

Patients with diabetes are at increased risk of developing diabetic nephropathy. This condition involves renal hypertrophy and hypertension and can eventually result in end-stage renal disease.

To reduce the patient's risk of developing nephropathy, teach him the importance of:

• avoiding frequent episodes of diabetic ketoacidosis

• avoiding the use of nephrotoxic agents

• controlling hypertension to slow the progression of diabetic nephropathy (decreases the rate at which the glomerular filtration rate declines)

• achieving and maintaining ideal body weight to help lower blood pressure

• recognizing and seeking treatment for urinary tract infections

• avoiding procedures that can lead to urinary tract infections, such as bladder catheterization in end-stage renal disease.

Neuropathy

Neuropathy occurs commonly among people with diabetes. To reduce the risk of developing neuropathy, teach the importance of:

• frequently examining the feet

Frequent examination of the feet is a must for preventing neuropathy.

• eliminating risk factors, such as smoking and hypertension
• immediately reporting symptoms of altered sensation, such as burning, tingling, or numbness
• maintaining meticulous foot care.

Cardiac complications

Intensive control of hypertension in people with type 2 diabetes significantly reduces the risk of heart failure, stroke, and death from other complications of diabetes. Stress the importance of maintaining normal blood pressure and tight blood glucose control to prevent cardiac complications.

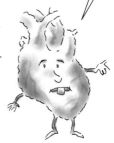

Controlling blood pressure is critical for cutting the risk of heart failure and stroke.

Quick quiz

1. Because undetected diabetes can have devastating consequences, laboratory screening is recommended for:
    A. adults over age 45.
    B. extremely thin individuals.
    C. pregnant women in their first trimester.

Answer: A. Laboratory screening is recommended for adults over age 45, obese individuals, pregnant women during the 24th to 28th week of gestation, women with a history of obstetric complications or gestational diabetes, women who delivered a baby weighing over 9 lb (4.1 kg), patients with impaired glucose tolerance, and patients with reactive hypoglycemia.

2. A high-fiber diet can protect against the development of diabetes by:
  A. slowing carbohydrate absorption.
  B. causing more rapid elimination of carbohydrates and proteins.
  C. enhancing the body's counter-regulatory response to high blood glucose.

Answer: A. Fiber protects against diabetes by slowing carbohydrate absorption, thus reducing demand on the pancreas to produce insulin.

3. A patient with diabetes who smokes is at higher risk for limb amputation because smoking:

    A. reduces skin sensation.

    B. causes peripheral vasoconstriction.

    C. leads to neuronal inflammation in joints.

Answer: B. Smoking alters peripheral circulation by constricting blood vessels and compromising cells distal to the constriction.

4. For a patient with diabetes, weight control is critical because obesity causes:

    A. insulin resistance.

    B. beta cell destruction.

    C. increased glycogenolysis.

Answer: A. Obesity is a major cause of insulin resistance. Controlling weight plays a key role in controlling blood glucose levels and can also help reverse impaired glucose tolerance in obese diabetics.

Scoring

☆☆☆   If you answered all four questions correctly, jump for joy! You passed your screen test with amazing success! Oh, Mr. DeMille? She's ready for her close-up!

☆☆   If you answered three questions correctly, super! You made it through the initial screening process. We've got our eye on you!

☆   If you answered fewer than three questions correctly, not to worry. You'll get a screening room call-back for sure!

3

Assessing patients with diabetes

Key facts
♦ Diabetes affects every system in the body.
♦ In addition to high blood glucose levels, several classic signs confirm the diagnosis of diabetes, including the three P's — polydipsia, polyphagia, and polyuria.
♦ Many patients with type 2 diabetes first seek medical care as a result of advanced systemic effects of diabetes.
♦ Within 10 years of onset, half of all patients with diabetes have retinopathy that may progress to blindness.

When you suspect diabetes

Assessment of a person suspected of having diabetes involves a number of procedures, including:
• taking a thorough health history
• conducting an in-depth physical examination
• performing a variety of diagnostic tests, as indicated.

Advice from the experts

Speed of onset

Note the severity and duration of the patient's complaints, which may help identify the type of diabetes involved.
- Type 1 diabetes usually causes pronounced, rapidly developing symptoms.
- Type 2 diabetes usually leads to vague, long-standing symptoms that develop gradually.

A diagnosis of diabetes involves a health history, physical examination, and numerous diagnostic tests.

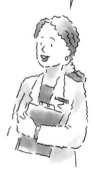

Focus on findings

During your assessment, focus on identifying signs and symptoms:
- directly related to elevated blood glucose levels
- arising from long-term effects of elevated blood glucose levels
- resulting from disease processes accelerated or exacerbated by diabetes.

Health history

Begin your assessment by obtaining a thorough history. Pay particular attention to the patient's initial complaint. (See *Speed of onset.*)

P, P, and — oh, yes — P

The patient with diabetes typically complains of one or more of these classic symptoms before diagnosis:

• polydipsia (excessive thirst) from polyuria-induced dehydration

• polyphagia (excessive hunger) from increased metabolic needs caused by tissue destruction

• polyuria (excessive urination) as a result of osmotic diuresis caused by excessive blood glucose.

From the 3 P's to...

The patient with diabetes may experience weight loss and fatigue resulting from loss of carbohydrate fuel and fat and protein depletion to satisfy energy needs. (Weight loss and fatigue commonly occur among people with unrecognized diabetes.)

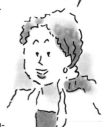

If your patient urinates large amounts frequently and is overly thirsty and hungry, suspect diabetes.

Memory jogger

To remember the three P's of diabetes (polydipsia, polyphagia, and polyuria), think of three people named Polly — one drinking, one eating, and one running for the nearest bathroom.

The patient may also complain of:

- dry, itchy skin
- frequent skin infections (such as boils, carbuncles, or furuncles)
- vaginal discomfort or irritation
- vision changes
- weakness.

Past medical history

Ask the patient about past conditions that may be associated with diabetes. In particular, note factors that can increase blood glucose levels, including:

- autoimmune dysfunction
- certain other endocrine disorders, particularly thyroid or adrenal disease
- delivery of an infant weighing more than 9 lb (4.1 kg)
- family history of diabetes, especially type 2
- history of gestational diabetes
- recent stress
- recent steroid use
- recent viral infection.

Socioeconomic history

When you investigate a patient's socioeconomic history, remember to assess:

- culture

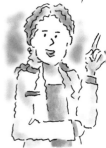

Remember to find out about the patient's past and present health as well as his socioeconomic history.

- dietary habits
- economic factors
- educational factors
- exercise history
- general physical condition
- growth and development of children
and adolescents
- lifestyle
- nutritional status
- psychosocial factors
- risk factors for atherosclerosis.

Physical findings

Perform a thorough physical examination
to identify signs and complications of diabetes. (See *Assessing previously diagnosed
diabetics,* page 58.) Keep in mind that the
effects of diabetes may occur even in a patient unaware of the disease. A complete
physical examination includes assessment of the eyes, skin, and vascular, renal, nervous, and immune systems.

Eyes

Early retinal changes may not cause
symptoms but may be detected on eye
examination. An ophthalmoscopic exami-

Advice from the experts

Assessing previously diagnosed diabetics

If the patient has already been diagnosed with diabetes, determine and review the following:

- how well he understands the disease
- what problems he has encountered
- how successfully he has managed his disease
- whether he has medical insurance that will cover diabetic supplies such as insulin, insulin syringe, and glucometer
- whether he has noticed symptoms of complications
- details of previous treatment programs, including nutrition and diabetes self-management training
- current treatment, including medications, meal plans, and results of glucose monitoring
- frequency of complications, such as ketoacidosis and hypoglycemia
- medications that may affect blood glucose levels.

Key signs

In addition, assess and review:

- prior glycohemoglobin A_{1C} levels
- presence of skin, foot, dental, or genitourinary (GU) infections
- signs of chronic complications of the eyes; the kidneys; the nervous, GU, and GI systems; the heart; and peripheral vascular and cerebrovascular function.

nation and pupil dilatation is necessary to fully assess for early retinal changes.

Microvascular changes

Eye changes in a patient with diabetes result primarily from microvascular retinal changes. Early changes include retinal microaneurysm, followed by microinfarction and exudate formation.

Proliferative retinopathy

These early changes may progress to proliferative retinopathy, a serious condition characterized by the formation of new blood vessels in the retina (neovascularization). Eventually, retinal detachment and vitreous hemorrhage may occur. Within 10 years of disease onset, half of all patients with diabetes have some degree of diabetic retinopathy, a condition that may progress rapidly to blindness.

Skin

Skin changes, especially on the legs and feet, result from neuropathies and from microvascular and macrovascular changes.

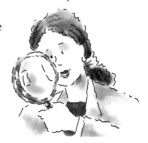

Examine the patient's skin closely, particularly on his legs and feet.

Your skin's showing

• Examine the patient's skin closely, particularly on his legs and feet.

• Look for lesions and infections that might have developed in corns, calluses, hypertrophied skin, or ingrown toenails. (See *Gangrene and other lesions*.)

• Check for gangrene (due to changes in blood vessels and decreased peripheral sensation), a condition significantly more common in patients with diabetes than in people who don't have diabetes.

• Remember to document your findings and to stress the need for proper foot care.

Vascular system

Because vascular changes may be microvascular or macrovascular, make sure to carefully assess the patient's peripheral pulses and blood pressure. Checking these signs in several body positions helps paint a clear picture of the extent of vascular changes.

Microvascular changes

Microvascular changes are characterized by a thickened, damaged capillary base-

Warning!

Gangrene and other lesions

Gangrene may stem from minor trauma or an undetected infection caused by sensory nerve loss. Gangrene may be dry (not involving an infection) or wet (associated with an infection). Report signs of gangrene immediately; the patient may require amputation.

Other lesions

Also assess for such abnormal skin lesions as:
• neurotrophic ulcer, an insensitive lesion typically developing under corns and calluses. Such a lesion may progress to infection with bone involvement.
• reddish-brown papular spots called diabetic dermopathy. This condition may progress to crusts and scar tissue.
• ulcerating necrotic processes, called necrobiosis lipoidica. These plaquelike lesions, which have a yellowish center and brown border, may progress to ulceration. These lesions are found in less than 1% of people with diabetes and most heal with aggressive local care.

ment membrane, especially in uncontrolled diabetes. Clinical effects include:
• atherosclerosis
• hypertension

• increased risk for lipid disorders, particularly hyperlipoproteinemia
• nephropathy
• retinopathy
• skin changes. (See *Acute and chronic complications*.)

Macrovascular changes

Macrovascular changes occur in people with type 2 diabetes and appear as atherosclerotic changes in blood vessels. These changes are unrelated to the

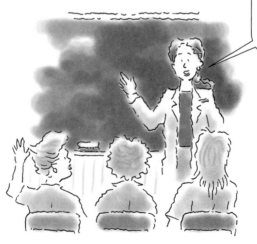

Your nurse will check your pulses and blood pressure in different positions as part of your physical examination.

Warning!

Acute and chronic complications

Because diabetes causes widespread effects, your review of all body systems provides key assessment data. If you note signs of acute complications, notify the primary care provider and begin interventions as directed.

Acute complications

- Cardiovascular disease
- Diabetic ketoacidosis
- Hyperosmolar hyperglycemic nonketotic syndrome
- Hypoglycemia

Chronic complications

- Nephropathy
- Neuropathy
- Peripheral vascular disease
- Retinopathy

severity of diabetes; patients with diabetes tend to develop the condition at an earlier age and have more extensive and rapidly progressing disease than do nondiabetics. Evidence suggest that hyperinsulinemia plays an important role in the development of macrovascular changes, the leading cause of death in patients with diabetes.

What's behind macrovascular changes?

Macrovascular changes are due to:
• decreased high-density lipoprotein levels
• development of fibrous plaques
• elevated serum cholesterol levels
• presence of lipid deposits in plaques.

People with diabetes are prone to develop a number of cardiovascular disorders.

All those changes can lead to...

Large-vessel atherosclerosis can compromise tissue oxygenation, contributing to the development of:
• cerebrovascular disease
• coronary artery disease
• peripheral vascular disease
• renal stenosis.

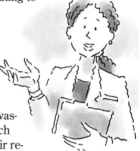

Renal system

Nephropathy results from microvascular changes in the kidneys. Such changes may progressively impair renal function. Renal changes may include:
• arteriosclerosis of the renal arteries or afferent or efferent arterioles
• glomerular lesions
• tubular lesions.

Check those labs

During your assessment of the renal system, check laboratory data for:

• proteinuria, an early sign of a glomerular lesion

• increased serum creatinine and blood urea nitrogen levels. These signs, along with oliguria, may indicate renal insufficiency, which can progress to renal failure.

Neuropathy can occur in any area of the nervous system. It's a head-to-toe kind of thing.

Nervous system

Diabetes affects the entire nervous system and can cause a number of neuropathies. Neurologic changes may take place in the peripheral, autonomic, or central nervous systems.

Talk about your wide variety

Neuropathy can cause widely varying signs and symptoms:

• Peripheral neuropathies may affect sensory and motor function, with sensory fibers usually affected first.

• Autonomic nervous system neuropathies may cause gastric motility changes, incontinence, or impotence.
• Neuropathies that stem from metabolic changes may lead to sorbitol accumulation in nerve cells and in fluid shifts, followed by cell swelling, rupture, and destruction.
• Peripheral neuropathy, which starts as diminished sensation, can progress to paresthesia and motor nerve involvement.

Immune system

Patients with diabetes are also at increased risk for infection and are frequently more susceptible to it. Assess the oral cavity and ask about dental infections. Other common infections to assess for include acute pyelonephritis, candidiasis, *Staphylococcus* skin infections, and vaginitis.

Children and adolescents

Assessment of children and adolescents who might have diabetes requires additional steps. When performing a physical examination on a child or adolescent, determine the patient's:

• height and weight measurement and
compare them to normal measurements
for their age range
• sexual maturation (in prepubertal patients)
• blood pressure compared to age-
related norms.

Diagnostic tests

A diagnosis of diabetes is based on the
patient's symptoms plus a casual plasma
glucose concentration of 200 mg/dl or
higher. A casual plasma glucose value is
one that's obtained any time of the day,
regardless of the time of the patient's
most recent meal.

More tests

For any test, questionable results should
be confirmed by repeating tests on a different day. More frequent testing is recommended for high-risk groups. Other
laboratory tests that can aid in the diagnosis of diabetes include:
• fasting glucose level, normally below
126 mg/dl. To obtain a fasting value, the
patient should have had no caloric intake
for at least 8 hours.

Testing for gestational diabetes

The recommended screening test for a patient with gestational diabetes mellitus (GDM) involves a modified glucose tolerance test, with oral administration of 50 g of glucose, called a glucose challenge or glucose load. If the blood glucose level is 150 mg/dl or higher 1 hour after the glucose challenge, a full glucose tolerance test with an oral glucose load of 100 g is performed.

Confirming the diagnosis

GDM is confirmed if two blood glucose levels are at or above:

- 105 mg/dl in the fasting state
- 190 mg/dl 1 hour after ingestion
- 165 mg/dl 2 hours after ingestion
- 145 mg/dl 3 hours after ingestion.

• oral glucose tolerance test, the most sensitive method of evaluating borderline cases of diabetes. (See *Testing for gestational diabetes.*) Blood and urine glucose levels are monitored for up to 6 hours after ingestion of a challenge dose of 75 to 100 g of glucose.

Quick quiz

1. Classic symptoms of diabetes include:

    A. excessive thirst, hunger, and urination.

    B. pallor, excessive sweating, and constipation.

    C. weakness, a sweet taste in the mouth, and dizziness.

Answer: A. Classic symptoms of diabetes include polydipsia (excessive thirst), polyphagia (excessive hunger), and polyuria (excessive urination) — the three P's of diabetes.

2. Past conditions that may be associated with diabetes include:

    A. delivery of an infant weighing under 5 lb (2.25 kg).

    B. history of cardiomegaly or other cardiovascular condition.

    C. history of Cushing's syndrome or other endocrine imbalance.

Answer: C. Past conditions that may be associated with diabetes include autoimmune dysfunction, other endocrine disorders (particularly thyroid or adrenal disease), delivery of an infant weighing more than 9 lb (4.1 kg), family history of diabetes (especially type 2), history of gestational diabetes mellitus, recent stress, recent use of steroids, or recent viral infection.

3. Retinal changes in a patient with diabetes result primarily from:

    A. lipid deposits on the retina.

    B. macrovascular damage.

    C. microvascular damage.

Answer: C. Eye changes in a patient with diabetes result primarily from microvascular retinal changes.

Scoring

☆☆☆ If you answered all three questions correctly, wowsa! Our assessment is in: There's no stopping your success!

☆☆ If you answered two questions correctly, ooh-la-la! Our diagnosis is clear: Your knowledge is expanding exponentially.

☆ If you answered fewer than two questions correctly, not to fret. Assess your responses, and take steps to prevent further complications.

4

Treating patients with diabetes

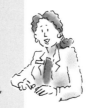

Key facts
- ◆ Treatment for diabetes typically includes diet, exercise, and insulin therapy or oral antidiabetic drugs.
- ◆ A wide variety of delivery devices can be used to administer insulin, including pens, indwelling catheters, and pumps.
- ◆ Certain patients with diabetes may benefit from islet cell transplantation.

Treatment overview

Treatment goals for patients with diabetes include:
- preventing long-term complications
- ensuring normal psychosocial adaptation
- helping to normalize carbohydrate, fat, and protein metabolism
- avoiding hypoglycemia and other treatment-related complications.

Type 1...

The primary treatment for a patient with type 1 diabetes is insulin, an essential drug for managing diabetes. Other treatments include dietary measures and exercise. If your patient develops insulin resistance, his primary care provider may add an oral antidiabetic drug.

...Type 2

For patients with type 2 diabetes, treatments generally include dietary measures, an exercise program, and antidiabetic drugs or insulin therapy.

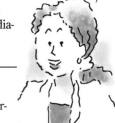

Type 1 patients usually receive insulin. Most type 2 patients can be managed on oral antidiabetic drugs alone.

Diet

Because diet is the body's most important source of glucose, diet is considered the cornerstone of care. (See *Eating right*.) Your patient must carefully monitor his food intake to prevent widely fluctuating blood glucose levels.

Advice from the experts

Eating right

The American Diabetes Association (ADA) has established dietary guidelines for the patient with diabetes. This chart notes the ideal percentage of the patient's daily intake for each element. (In addition to these elements, the ADA recommends that the patient eat 20 to 35 g of fiber per day.)

Element	Percentage of daily intake
Protein	10% to 20%
Carbohydrates and monounsaturated fats	60% to 70%
Saturated fats	less than 10%
Polyunsaturated fats	up to 10%

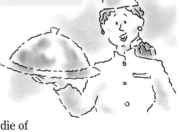

Try a low-calorie diet for your diabetes. It will reduce your body's need for insulin.

Risk of high cholesterol

At least 50% of Americans with diabetes have increased cholesterol levels, and 75% Americans with diabetes die of heart disease. Patients with diabetes also face a higher than average risk of recurrent myocardial infarction.

Patients with type 2 diabetes face an even greater risk because many have lipoprotein abnormalities. These abnormalities include overproduction of very-low-density lipoproteins (VLDL), defective lipolysis of VLDL triglycerides, and normal levels of low-density lipoproteins (LDL), a condition known as type IV hyperlipidemia.

Did you know that having either type 1 or type 2 diabetes puts me at increased risk for heart disease? I sure didn't.

Cutting that cholesterol

The good news is that a reduction in cholesterol levels, even those that are mildly or moderately elevated, can reduce the incidence of cardiac disease by up to 50%. What's more, a class of drugs, 3-hydroxy-3-methylglutaryl coenzyme A (HMG-CoA) reductase inhibitors (sometimes called statins), may help ward off early onset heart disease in patients with type 2 diabetes. By inhibiting the enzyme that controls cholesterol production, these drugs reduce the levels of both VLDL and LDL cholesterol.

Long on legumes

A high fiber intake seems to help control blood glucose levels and blood lipid concentrations. A diet high in fiber may delay gastric emptying and slow digestion and absorption. The American Diabetes Association now recommends 20 to 35 g of fiber a day. Encourage the patient to eat such high-fiber foods as bran cereals, fresh fruits, fresh vegetables, and legumes.

Nothing simple about sugar intake

Discuss the effects of concentrated sweets (foods high in simple sugars) with your patient. Sources include ice cream, soft drinks, juice, cookies, pastries, and candies. The body absorbs these concentrated sweets much more quickly than complex carbohydrates. The result is a rapid rise in blood glucose levels.

Foods are now categorized according to their glycemic index, meaning the blood glucose level after ingestion of the food. (See *Using the glycemic index,* page 76.) Believe it or not, baked potatoes have a higher glycemic index than ice cream.

Using the glycemic index

Researchers now categorize carbohydrates according to the blood glucose level each one produces after ingestion. They assign a rating called the glycemic index to each food. Foods with a low glycemic index don't cause a rapid increase in blood glucose levels, while those with a higher glycemic index do. The index is designed to help patients minimize increases in blood glucose levels.

As food becomes more processed, it enters the bloodstream as glucose more quickly. That's why eating a baked potato or a whole piece of fruit is better for a person with diabetes rather than eating mashed potatoes or drinking fruit juice. Likewise, bread has a higher glycemic index than pasta.

Exercise

Exercise can lower blood glucose levels without the administration of additional insulin. Exercise is not a complete remedy for diabetes, but it's a vital part of your patient's treatment regimen. To help your patient implement an exercise plan, do the following:

• Make sure that he has had a preexercise evaluation by his primary care provider to identify previously undiagnosed problems, such as hypertension and silent ischemic heart disease.

• Help him choose an aerobic exercise, such as walking, running, cycling, or swimming.

• Tell him that the cardiovascular benefits of exercise are important for lowering his risk of cardiovascular disease. (See *Anaerobic exercise and diabetes,* page 78.)

Ride the wave. Use exercise to help lower blood glucose levels.

Going to the gym?

When reviewing your patient's workout regimen, remember to tell him to:

• build up to exercising at least three times a week on alternate days, with each session lasting between 45 and 60 minutes

• check his blood glucose level before and after exercising and avoid exercise if his blood glucose level is below 250 mg/dl

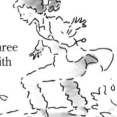

Advice from the experts

Anaerobic exercise and diabetes

Tell your patient to avoid anaerobic exercise, such as weight lifting or push-ups. Anaerobic exercise doesn't use glucose as fuel. Consequently, the exercise-induced stress can cause an increase in blood glucose levels. Anaerobic exercise also causes a rapid heart rate and an increase in blood pressure, both of which could be dangerous for a patient prone to cardiovascular disease.

- carry quick-acting carbohydrates when exercising, to treat hypoglycemia
- stop exercising if he gets dizzy
- drink water before, during, and after exercise to maintain hydration
- inject insulin in a site other than near muscles that will receive the most exercise during activity
- check his feet before and after exercise; foot injuries can occur with high-impact exercise
- wear well-cushioned shoes with white protective socks to help prevent skin infections on the foot.

Hitting the target

Teach your patient that he should exercise enough to reach his target heart rate. To determine the target heart rate, subtract the patient's age from 220, and then multiply the result by 0.7. Warn your patient never to exceed his target heart rate while exercising.

Insulin therapy

Insulin therapy may be prescribed alone or in combination with oral antidiabetic drugs, depending on the patient's hypoglycemia pattern. Insulin therapy aims to alleviate hyperglycemia, while at the same time avoiding hypoglycemia.

Insulin: Gotta have it

A patient with type 1 diabetes needs insulin to properly use the glucose he receives from meals. In addition to insulin's role in glucose metabolism, the hormone is also essential for normalizing blood glucose levels. If he has an absolute deficiency of insulin, he'll need insulin replacement to survive.

Insulin for acute stress

If hyperglycemia in a patient with type 2 diabetes is unresponsive to diet and exercise, the patient will need oral antidiabetic drugs. Occasionally, a patient with type 2 diabetes will also need insulin. For a patient with type 2 diabetes experiencing a period of acute stress — for example, surgery or acute illness — blood glucose levels may increase temporarily and insulin may be required for a time.

Types of insulin

Insulin can be categorized by its origin (beef, pork, or human), purity (standard or purified), or duration of action. (See *Available insulins*.) Duration of action categories for insulin are:
• ultra-short acting (onset, 15 minutes; duration, 1 hour)
• short-acting (onset, 30 to 60 minutes; duration, 5 to 8 hours)
• intermediate-acting (onset, 1 to 2 hours; duration, 18 to 24 hours)
• long-acting (onset, 4 to 6 hours; duration, 24 to 36 hours)

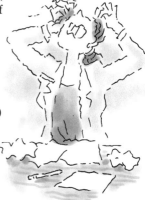

Stressed out? You may need to increase your insulin dosage temporarily.

Battling illness

Available insulins

The insulins now available are divided into standard and purified categories and then into rapid-acting, intermediate-acting, and long-acting subcategories. This chart highlights key insulins in each category, their manufacturer, and species of origin.

Trade name	Manufacturer	Origin
Standard		
Rapid-acting		
Humalog	Lilly	Human
Regular Iletin I	Lilly	Beef or pork
Regular Iletin II	Novo Nordisk	Pork
Intermediate-acting		
NPH Iletin I	Lilly	Beef or pork
Lente Iletin I	Lilly	Beef or pork
NPH Insulin	Novo Nordisk	Beef
Lente Insulin	Novo Nordisk	Beef
Long-acting		
Ultralente U	Novo Nordisk	Beef
Purified		
Rapid-acting		
Regular Purified Pork Insulin Injection	Novo Nordisk	Pork
Velosulin	Novo Nordisk	Human
Humulin R	Lilly	Human
Novolin R	Novo Nordisk	Human

(continued)

Available insulins (continued)

Trade name	Manufacturer	Origin
Purified (continued)		
Intermediate-acting		
NPH-N	Novo Nordisk	Pork
Lente L	Novo Nordisk	Pork
Humulin 70/30	Lilly	Human
Humulin L	Lilly	Human
Humulin N	Lilly	Human
Novolin L	Novo Nordisk	Human
Novolin 70/30	Novo Nordisk	Human
Novolin N	Novo Nordisk	Human
Long-acting		
Humulin U, Ultralente	Lilly	Human

• mixtures (onset, ½ hour to 2½ hours; duration, 14 to 24 hours).

Mixing Lente and regular: A no-no

Regular insulin shouldn't be mixed with an intermediate-acting insulin that contains zinc, such as Lente Iletin I, Lente Insulin, or Lente L. The zinc ions in the intermediate-acting insulin will bind with the regular insulin and delay its action. If regular insulin must be mixed with a zinc-containing insulin, the injection should be given immediately after or within 15 minutes of mixing to prevent the binding of excess zinc with regular insulin, thus delaying insulin's actions.

Before the first course

Humalog, the newest human insulin analog, is similar to regular insulin except for its chemical makeup. (The placement of the amino acids lysine and proline are reversed.) Humalog works more quickly than regular insulin, allowing it to be administered immediately before a meal.

Prescribing insulin

Primary health care providers consider two factors when prescribing insulin: purity and cost. Purer insulins cause fewer insulin allergies, less insulin resistance, and less lipodystrophy. However, purer insulins also cost more. Human insulin is generally the purest — but also most expensive — insulin prescribed.

When pork and beef are off the menu

The American Diabetes Association recommends human (rather than pork or beef) insulin for use in:
- pregnant women
- women considering pregnancy

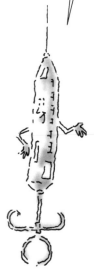

Before you take a bite, take a hit of Humalog to cover the "eats" to come!

- patients beginning insulin therapy
- patients expected to use insulin intermittently only
- individuals with allergies or immune resistance to animal-derived insulin.

Delivering insulin

A patient typically requires daily injections of insulin, but the primary care provider may prescribe insulin several times a day. (See *Teaching about insulin.*) In addition to a conventional syringe, other devices are available for delivering insulin. These devices include:

- external insulin pumps

You needn't worry about injecting yourself with a regular syringe. Special pumps and even insulin pens are now available.

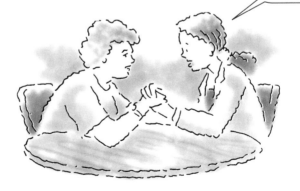

Teaching about insulin

When your patient is taking insulin, teach him to:
- keep spare bottles of each type of insulin refrigerated
- keep the current bottle of insulin at room temperature
- inspect the bottle before each use for clumping, precipitation, or change in clarity or color and not use the bottle if he sees these characteristics
- roll the insulin vial between his palms to ensure uniformity of solution
- draw up regular insulin first when mixing regular insulin with NPH
- avoid mixing regular insulin and Lente insulin
- rotate anatomic injection sites
- use proper injection technique, including infection control procedures and proper needle disposal
- time his meals to correspond to the onset and peak times of insulin therapy
- carry at least 15 g of a fast-acting carbohydrate that can be eaten quickly if he has a hypoglycemic reaction
- carry important medical information on a bracelet or wallet card, alerting people that he's taking insulin.

- indwelling subcutaneous catheters
- inhaled insulin
- insulin jet injectors
- insulin patch
- insulin pens
- programmable implantable medication system (PIMS).

Fashionable accessory

External insulin pumps provide continuous subcutaneous insulin infusion. They can deliver insulin in basal (small) doses every few minutes or in bolus (large) doses that the patient sets manually. The pump system consists of a reservoir containing regular insulin, a small pump, an infusion rate selector, a battery, and a plastic catheter with an attached needle leading from the syringe to the subcutaneous injection site.

The infusion rate selector automatically releases half the total daily insulin requirement. The patient releases the remainder in bolus amounts before meals and snacks. The patient can fasten the pump to his belt or slip it into his pocket. The patient must change the syringe daily and change the needle, catheter, and injection site every other day.

New research indicates that using an external pump, with very short-acting insulin, can give patients the tightest blood glucose control with the least risk of hypoglycemia.

For frequent injections

An indwelling subcutaneous catheter can benefit a patient needing frequent injections because it allows him to inject insulin through a catheter port. The device features an 18-mm catheter and port over a 24G 19-mm needle. The catheter can be used for 3 to 7 days. The patient inserts the device into the subcutaneous tissue of his abdomen and then withdraws the needle, leaving the catheter in place.

> For patients needing a quick burst of insulin, you almost can't beat an insulin inhaler.

Take a deep breath

The use of inhaled insulin is being investigated. Drawing from a device the size of a flashlight, the patient can inhale a fine powder form of a short-acting insulin. The powder is rapidly absorbed into the bloodstream.

But does it help you quit smoking?

An insulin patch applied to the skin can deliver a continuous low dose of insulin. The patient can pull off a tab on the patch to release extra insulin before meals. This mode of delivery is still being studied.

Quick but expensive

With insulin jet injectors, insulin is delivered through a high-pressure air mechanism. Insulin jet injectors can disperse insulin fast and promote absorption rapidly because they avoid the "puddling effect" common to regular injections. However, they're expensive and require disposable needles.

Just don't try to write with it

An insulin pen, which looks like an ordinary writing instrument, typically contains a cartridge that holds 100 to 200 U of insulin. The patient can select the dosage by turning a dial on the pen. The device features a needle end, which the patient holds against his skin, and a plunger end, which the patient presses to deliver the insulin.

Insulin pens are recommended for those taking three or more doses of insulin a day. They're easy for the patient to carry, and visually impaired patients may find dialing the dosage on an insulin pen easier than measuring an insulin dosage on a syringe.

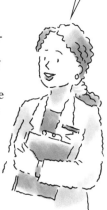

The insulin pen works great for patients needing three or more injections a day.

AM or FM?

Weighing 6 to 8 oz (170 to 227 g) and sur-gically implanted (usually on the left side of the abdomen), the PIMS consists of a disk-shaped pump unit and a catheter. The pump holds and delivers the insulin. The catheter feeds the insulin directly into the peritoneal cavity.

The pump, encased in a titanium shell, contains a tiny computer that regulates the insulin dosage. The computer runs on a battery that typically lasts about 5 years.

The patient uses a small, hand-held external radio transmitter to control insulin release from the pump. Because the PIMS doesn't have a built-in blood glucose sen-sor, the patient must record his blood glucose levels several times daily to keep track of in-sulin requirements.

Lightweight and program-mable, the insulin pump is great for diabetics on the go.

Complications of insulin therapy

Complications associated with insulin therapy include:
• hypoglycemia
• insulin lipodystrophy caused by contin-uously using the same injection site

- insulin allergy
- insulin resistance
- irritation at the site, which is usually caused by cold insulin.

Somogyi what?

Another complication of insulin therapy is the Somogyi phenomenon. The Somogyi phenomenon occurs when hypoglycemia is followed by a compensatory period of rebound hyperglycemia as the body increases glucose production to correct the problem. Typically, the Somogyi phenomenon occurs during the late night or early morning when the patient is asleep.

During this time, insulin continues to be absorbed from the subcutaneous injection site, though insufficient glucose may be present for insulin to act. As a result, the blood glucose level drops rapidly. In response, the body secretes glucagon, norepinephrine, and corticosteroids to correct the hypoglycemia.

Although the patient awakens with symptoms of hyperglycemia, the earli-

> Rebound hyperglycemia, or the Somogyi phenomenon, most commonly occurs late at night.

er hypoglycemia is the condition that
must be corrected to prevent recurrence.

Therapy with oral antidiabetic drugs

Oral antidiabetic drugs are typically used
for patients with stable type 2 diabetes.
Some primary care providers prescribe
oral drugs along with insulin for patients
with type 1 diabetes who have severe insulin resistance.

The pancreas must be at least minimally functional for an oral antidiabetic drug to work properly.

How they work

Generally accepted theory suggests that
oral antidiabetic drugs produce pancreatic and extrapancreatic actions to regulate
blood glucose levels. These drugs probably stimulate pancreatic beta cells
to release insulin. The pancreas already must be functioning at a
minimal level.

Within a few weeks to a
few months of the initial response to a sulfonylurea, the
most commonly used family of
oral drugs, insulin secretion
drops to pretreatment levels.
However, blood glucose levels re-
main normal or near-normal.

Extrapancreatic actions of oral antidiabetic drugs probably maintain this continued control of blood glucose levels.

Why add a second oral drug?

Use of just one antidiabetic drug alone increases the risk of weight gain and hypoglycemia. Therefore, many people with diabetes take two or more drugs. The primary care provider determines the patient's particular response to the antidiabetic drug using a 2-week diary that includes the results of the patient's daily blood glucose levels, diet, symptoms, and exercise pattern. (See *Teaching about oral antidiabetic drugs*.) The four classes of oral antidiabetic drugs now available include:

• alpha glucosidase inhibitors (used for patients with high postprandial blood glucose levels)

• biguanides (used for patients with an overproduction of glucose in the liver)

• sulfonylureas (used for patients with insufficient insulin production)

• thiazolidinediones (used for patients with insulin resistance).

> Of the four classes of oral antidiabetic drugs, sulfonylureas are used most often.

Listen up!

Teaching about oral antidiabetic drugs

Teach your patient taking an oral antidiabetic drug about:
- the drug's action
- adverse reactions and when to call the primary care provider
- hypoglycemia's signs and symptoms and appropriate interventions if they occur.

Other instructions

Also tell the patient:
- that the drug doesn't replace dietary measures but works with them to help control blood glucose levels
- to take the drug only as ordered and never to alter the frequency or dose without consulting the primary care provider
- to continue taking the drug because uncontrolled hyperglycemia might result otherwise.

Complications of oral drugs

Possible complications that can occur from taking oral antidiabetic drugs include hypoglycemia and hyperglycemia as well as drug-specific adverse reactions including allergic reaction. In addition, certain patients should never take oral antidiabetic drugs. (See *When oral drugs shouldn't be used,* page 94.)

Before you give that drug

When oral drugs shouldn't be used

Some patients with diabetes shouldn't be given an oral antidiabetic drug, including patients who:

- are pregnant or breast-feeding
- are allergic to elements of the drug
- have severe renal or hepatic disease
- have diabetic ketoacidosis.

Transplantation

For a select group of patients with diabetes, transplantation of the pancreas or islet cells may be the best way to gain control of blood glucose levels. These transplants can free patients from the demands of self-administered insulin.

Following transplant surgery, the patient receives immunosuppressive therapy to prevent organ rejection.

Quick quiz

1. HMG-CoA reductase inhibitors work by:

    A. blocking the uptake of cholesterol in liver cells.

    B. increasing the rate of excretion of cholesterol.

    C. inhibiting the enzyme that controls cholesterol production.

Answer: C. HMG-CoA reductase inhibitors (sometimes called statins) may help ward off early onset heart disease in patients with type 2 diabetes. By inhibiting the enzyme that controls cholesterol production, these drugs reduce the levels of both VLDL and LDL cholesterol.

2. Because Humalog works more quickly than regular insulin, the drug is commonly administered:

    A. 1 hour before a meal.

    B. immediately before a meal.

    C. 1 hour after a meal.

Answer: B. Humalog works more quickly than regular insulin, allowing it to be administered immediately before a meal.

3. Oral antidiabetic drugs are *not* recommended for:

    A. patients who have type 2 diabetes.

    B. women who are pregnant or breast-feeding.

    C. patients who are allergic to insulin.

Answer: B. Pregnant or breast-feeding women should not receive oral antidiabetic drugs because the effects on the fetus and newborn haven't been determined.

Scoring

☆☆☆ If you answered all three questions correctly, yippee! You're our favorite Insulin Instructor!

☆☆ If you answered two of three questions correctly, too good! You can give us an injection of Humalog anytime!

☆ If you answered fewer than two questions correctly, s'no big deal. A bit of phenomenal Somogyi magic and you'll be back on top in no time!

5

Diabetes complications

Key facts
◆ Diabetes can lead to severe increases in blood glucose and ketoacid levels, causing significant complications.
◆ Early complications of diabetes include diabetic ketoacidosis, hyperosmolar hyperglycemic nonketotic syndrome, and hypoglycemia.
◆ Late complications affect every system of the body, with signs and symptoms varying depending on the system affected.

Early complications

Common early complications of diabetes include hypoglycemia, diabetic ketoacidosis (DKA), and hyperosmolar hyperglycemic nonketotic syndrome (HHNS). All of these complications can quickly cause death if the patient doesn't receive prompt assessment and treatment. (See *Reading the results*, page 99.)

Hypoglycemia

Although hypoglycemia — or insulin shock — can occur in people without diabetes, it's a particular risk for patients with diabetes. Hypoglycemia can result from delayed or missed meals, insulin overdose, or excessive exercise without adjustments in food intake or insulin use.

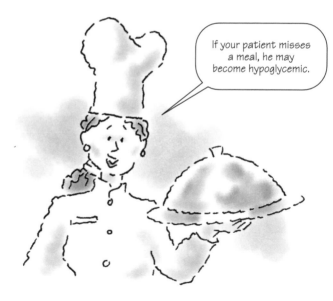

If your patient misses a meal, he may become hypoglycemic.

Reading the results

Discerning the difference between the main complications of diabetes — hypoglycemia, diabetic ketoacidosis (DKA), and hyperosmolar hyperglycemic nonketotic syndrome (HHNS) — can be difficult. This table of laboratory values will help you quickly assess your patient for these conditions.

Laboratory test	Hypoglycemia	DKA	HHNS
Arterial blood gas results	Normal or slight respiratory acidosis	Metabolic acidosis with compensatory respiratory alkalosis	Normal or slight metabolic acidosis
Blood glucose level	Below 70 mg/dl	250 to 800 mg/dl	Above 800 mg/dl
Hematocrit	Normal	Above normal	Above normal
Serum ketones	Normal	Greater than 80 mg/dl	Below 30 mg/dl
Serum osmolarity	Normal	Above normal but usually less than 330 mOsm/L	350 to 450 mOsm/L

(continued)

Reading the results *(continued)*

Laboratory test	Hypoglycemia	DKA	HHNS
Serum potassium level	Normal	Normal or above normal initially, then subnormal	Normal or above normal initially, then subnormal
Serum sodium level	Normal	Normal or subnormal	Above normal, normal, or subnormal
Urine glucose level	None	Above normal	Markedly above normal
Urine ketones	None	Positive or large amount present	Negative or small amount present
Urine output	Normal	*Initial* — polyuria *Late* — oliguria	Markedly above normal

Irritable and sweaty, then comatose

Hypoglycemia's onset varies from minutes to hours. Signs and symptoms include:
• cold, clammy skin

- hunger
- neurologic symptoms, including irritability, nervousness, giddiness, hand tremors, and difficulty with speaking, concentrating, focusing, and coordinating (early); hyperreflexia, dilated pupils, and coma (later)
- normal breath odor
- normal or above normal blood pressure
- normal or reduced muscle strength
- normal to rapid respirations early; bradypnea later
- pallor
- profuse sweating
- tachycardia (bradycardia in deep coma).

Diabetic ketoacidosis

DKA is triggered by extremely high glucose levels and usually occurs in patients with type 1 diabetes. This condition can result from undiagnosed diabetes, neglected treatment, infection, cardiovascular disorders, and physical or emotional stress.

It sneaks up on you

DKA's onset is slow, varying from hours to days. Its signs and symptoms include:
- abdominal pain
- anorexia
- crusty mucous membranes
- decreased bowel sounds
- deep and fast respirations (Kussmaul's respirations)
- extreme weakness
- fever (suggesting infection)
- fruity, acetone-like breath odor
- low blood pressure
- nausea or vomiting
- neurologic symptoms, including dullness, confusion, lethargy, and diminished reflexes (early); and coma (later)
- thirst
- warm, flushed, dry, and loose skin
- weak, rapid pulse
- weight loss.

A fruity odor to the breath is a sign of DKA.

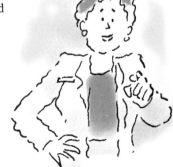

Hyperosmolar hyperglycemic nonketotic syndrome

HHNS, another acute complication of hyperglycemic crisis, usually occurs in patients with type 2 diabetes. This condition can result from undiagnosed diabetes, dehydration, infection, acute or chronic illness, certain drugs or medical procedures, or severe burns treated with high concentrations of glucose infusions.

Slow onset, quick signs

The onset of HHNS is slow — varying from hours to days — but occurs more rapidly than DKA. Signs and symptoms of HHNS are similar to that of DKA with three notable exceptions:

✌ Focal neurologic signs including hemiplegia commonly occur.

✌ Respirations are rapid but not deep.

✌ Breath odor is normal.

> If your patient has rapid, shallow breathing and focal deficits, think HHNS.

Late complications

Patients with diabetes can experience a number of systemic complications late in the disease. The most common late complications of diabetes include:

- cardiovascular and peripheral vascular disease
- nephropathy
- neuropathy
- retinopathy.

It's a mystery

Researchers aren't sure why these disorders are so prevalent among diabetics, but they do know that the complications usually appear about 10 years after the onset of diabetes. Researchers have also linked the incidence and severity of these complications to controlling blood glucose levels. Most primary care providers today advocate stringent control of blood glucose levels to minimize or prevent late complications.

> Tight glucose control is the order of the day for today's diabetes treatment.

Coronary and peripheral vascular diseases

Macrovascular changes from diabetes may cause coronary artery disease, cerebral vascular disease, or peripheral vascular disease. Treatment involves reducing the risk factors for coronary and peripheral vascular disease. The patient should:

- stop smoking
- control his hypertension
- reduce his cholesterol and triglyceride levels
- strictly control his blood glucose levels.

Nephropathy

Nephropathy, the result of microvascular changes in the kidneys, can lead to proteinuria, hypertension, edema, and renal insufficiency. Nephropathy can occur in patients who have had type 1 diabetes for 15 to 20 years. Of patients who develop nephropathy, nearly 40% eventually develop end-stage renal disease. Patients with type 2 diabetes tend to develop nephropathy within 5 to 10 years, with up to 5% of them eventually developing end-stage renal disease.

Unwanted place for protein

Protein in the urine is the first sign of kidney damage as a result of chronic hyperglycemia. If renal insufficiency develops, look for continued proteinuria, hypertension, elevated serum creatinine and blood urea nitrogen levels, and diminished glomerular filtration rate (25 to 30 ml/minute).

Signs and symptoms of uremia, which can occur in severe diabetes, include a glomerular filtration rate below 15 ml/minute, a serum creatinine level greater than 4 mg/dl, nausea, vomiting, lethargy, anemia, hypertension, and acidosis.

Take the burgers off the grill

Treatment for nephropathy involves placing the patient on a protein-restricted diet. For a patient with end-stage renal disease, a kidney transplant or dialysis may be needed.

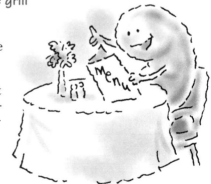

I'd like to order something from the low-protein side of the menu, please.

Neuropathy

Neuropathy, the result of microvascular changes in the neurons, can affect either the peripheral or autonomic nervous system. In this condition, myelin nerve fibers become demyelinated (which prevents the proper conduction of nerve impulses), connective tissues proliferate, and the capillary basement membrane thickens. The effects of the disorder depend on the particular nerves involved.

System by system

Autonomic neuropathy involves damage to one or more areas of the autonomic nervous system. Signs and symptoms depend on the particular system or organ affected:

• cardiovascular: orthostatic hypotension, mild but persistent tachycardia

• GI: gastroparesis resulting in delayed emptying of gastric contents, episodic diar-

> To function properly, I really need my beauty sheath.

rhea, retention of food, nausea, and vomiting
• genitourinary: urine retention, overflow incontinence, urinary tract infections, impotence, retrograde ejaculation, and inability to maintain erection
• sweat glands: episodic, profuse sweating.

Mono or poly?

The type of neuropathy is determined by the number of nerves involved. If one nerve is involved, the condition is termed mononeuropathy. The term distal symmetric polyneuropathy refers to a multiple-nerve neuropathy in a stocking-glove type of pattern, usually beginning at the toes and moving up over time to the calves. In most patients, by the time the neuropathy reaches the calves, a similar neuropathy has started at the fingertips before eventually moving up the arms.

Neuropathy signs and symptoms

Symptoms of neuropathy include numbness, tingling, burning, sudden pain in the area, a dull ache, and progressive cramping of the digits.

Symptoms worsen at night and may progress to a point that the patient can't tolerate pressure from the bed sheets. Muscle weakness, sensory loss, unbalanced gait, foot ulcers, and loss of fine motor skills occur with progression of the disease.

Treating the neuropathy

Treatment of neuropathy involves tight control of blood glucose levels to prevent further damage. Affected joints may be treated with splinting and, in some patients, corticosteroid injections. Recovery usually occurs within 3 months.

Medications may also be used to treat peripheral neuropathy and include nonsteroidal anti-inflammatory drugs, amitriptyline, topical capsaicin, or possibly an aldolase reductase inhibitor (currently under investigation). Surgery may also be required for patients with recurrent neuropathies such as carpal tunnel syndrome, a mononeuropathy.

Pain from neuropathy may be severe enough to require a steroid injection.

Retinopathy

Diabetic retinopathy, the result of microvascular changes in the eyes, is the leading cause of blindness in the United States. It's characterized by progressive deterioration of blood vessels in the retina and occurs in half of the patients who have had diabetes more than 10 years. About 9 out of 10 patients who don't control their blood glucose levels properly and are chronically hyperglycemic eventually develop retinopathy, which develops in three stages.

Retinopathy occurs in 90% of patients who control their diabetes poorly.

Stage one

Patients with stage one retinopathy (nonproliferative background) may experience no symptoms at all. By the time symptoms appear, the disease has often progressed to stage three, a more severe form of retinopathy. Patients who experience symptoms during stage one may exhibit:

• macular edema
• microaneurysms
• small intraretinal hemorrhages
• yellow lipid deposits (exudates).

Stage two

Stage two retinopathy (preproliferative) involves progression of stage one symptoms with occlusion of retinal capillaries, tortuous and bulging retinal veins, and the appearance of multiple blot hemorrhages. Cotton-wool spots may appear on examination.

Stage three

Stage three retinopathy (proliferative) involves growth of new and abnormal blood vessels on the retina, optic nerve, and iris. These vessels extend into the vitreous and easily hemorrhage. Fibrous scar tissue can form with retinal detachment. Loss of vision is generally the first sign. Suspect this stage if your patient complains of floating spots before his eyes, rapid visual changes, or fogged vision.

If a patient develops proliferative retinopathy, he may become blind.

Look to the laser

Treating retinopathy can involve laser photocoagulation, a procedure usually most beneficial when applied throughout the midperipheral retina. Vitreous hemorrhage is treated with removal of the vitreous.

Quick quiz

1. A complication of diabetes that may occur early in the disease is:

  A. DKA.

  B. nephropathy.

  C. neuropathy.

Answer: A. DKA is a slowly developing but serious complication of diabetes that can occur anytime but commonly occurs before a patient has been diagnosed with the disease.

2. Tremors, tachycardia, and cold, clammy skin are signs of:

  A. DKA.

  B. HHNS.

  C. hypoglycemia.

Answer: C. Tremors, tachycardia, and cold, clammy skin are all signs of hypoglycemia.

3. The first sign of kidney damage secondary to diabetes is:

  A. decreased urine output.

  B. elevated serum creatinine levels.

  C. proteinuria.

Answer: C. Proteinuria is the first sign of kidney damage. Decreased urine output and elevated serum creatinine levels occur later in the disease.

4. A patient whose joints are affected by neuropathy is typically treated with:
    A. a narcotic analgesic.
    B. splinting.
    C. ultrasound therapy.
Answer: B. Joints affected by neuropathy are commonly treated with splinting, nonsteroidal anti-inflammatory drugs, and capsaicin (and occasionally corticosteroid injections).

5. Stage three retinopathy (proliferative) is marked by the appearance of:
    A. macular edema and microaneurysms.
    B. retinal capillary occlusions, tortuous and bulging retinal veins, and multiple blot hemorrhages.
    C. growth of new and abnormal blood vessels on the retina, optic nerve, and iris.
Answer: C. Stage three retinopathy (proliferative) involves growth of new and abnormal blood vessels on the retina, optic nerve, and iris.

Scoring

★★★ If you answered all four questions correctly, excellent! You obviously didn't find this chapter on complications complicated.

★★ If you answered three questions correctly, very good! Your knowledge of early and late diabetic complications is remarkable.

★ If you answered fewer than three questions correctly, that's OK. Being a wonderful patient care provider means much more than just answering quiz questions correctly.

6

Teaching patients about diabetes

Key facts

♦ Patient education topics can vary widely, depending on how long your patient has had diabetes.

♦ Teaching your patient about late complications associated with diabetes may help him avoid them.

♦ Teaching the patient how hemoglobin A_{1c} levels can track blood glucose levels over time can help improve compliance.

♦ Proper skin and foot care may prevent serious complications.

Teaching strategies

As you teach your patient with diabetes, pay special attention to the way you present the information. Be positive, and help the patient feel empowered. If the patient feels he's in control of his diabetes, he will be more likely to believe that the changes he makes in his lifestyle will positively influence his condition.

Just the facts, please

Discuss the important aspects of diabetes with your newly diagnosed patient. Review with him:

• the changes that occur in the body as a result of diabetes and the reasons they occur

• acute complications of diabetes, such as diabetic ketoacidosis (DKA), hyperos-

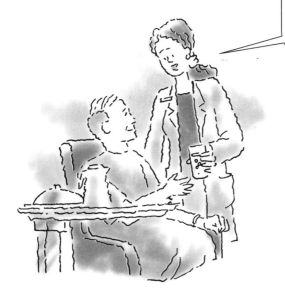

You can take charge of your diabetes. I'll be here to help in any way I can.

molar hyperglycemic nonketotic syndrome, and hypoglycemia
• the causes of acute complications and ways to avoid them
• late complications of diabetes and ways to prevent them.

Understanding blood glucose

Make sure your patient understands the differences between hypoglycemia and hyperglycemia.

Hypoglycemia

Explain that hypoglycemia may result from too much insulin, too little food, unusually strenuous exercise, or a delayed meal. Teach him that hypoglycemia's signs and symptoms include headache, excessive sweating, faintness, palpitations, trembling, impaired vision, hunger, irritability, and personality changes. Tell him to increase his blood glucose level by taking appropriate measures if he experiences any of these signs or symptoms.

Hyperglycemia

Explain that hyperglycemia may result from too little insulin, dietary noncompliance, infection, illness, or emotional distress. Explain that hyperglycemia's signs and symptoms include increased thirst; increased urination; weakness; abdominal pain; generalized aches; rapid, deep breathing (Kussmaul's respirations); nausea; and vomiting. Make sure that your patient knows the difference between hypoglycemia and hyperglycemia.

Advise the patient to call his primary care provider immediately if signs or symptoms of hyperglycemia appear, to take fluids without sugar if he can swallow, and to test

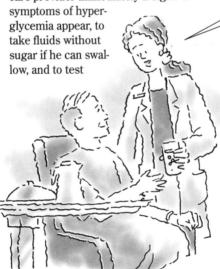

Sticking to your treatment program can help prevent episodes of hyperglycemia.

his blood glucose levels frequently. Most important, reassure him that he can prevent these episodes by adhering to his diet, drug therapy, exercise regimen, and sick-day guidelines.

Teaching about treatment

Review all therapies prescribed by the patient's primary care provider. Make sure that the patient understands each therapy, its purpose, benefits, and risks. Therapies might include drug therapy, exercise, diet, and home glucose monitoring as well as what to do if the patient becomes ill.

Drug therapy

Tell your patient the name, dosage, route, and adverse reactions of each drug. Make sure your patient understands that he should consult with his primary care provider before he takes a drug that wasn't prescribed for him. Review administration information for each drug, including insulin or oral antidiabetic drugs.

Insulin instruction

If your patient has been prescribed insulin, review the type of insulin and the way to inject it. Make sure he can read the number of units and can inject them properly. In addition, review the:

• purpose of insulin and its timing with meals

• way he should travel with insulin

• need for changing injection sites. For example, he might use eight places on the abdomen 1 week, and four places on the thigh the next.

> Special products are available for a patient who can't read the markings on a syringe.

Oral antidiabetic drugs

If your patient has been prescribed an oral antidiabetic drug, review the purpose of the drug and the way it will affect his diabetes. Discuss the timing of dosages and meals. In addition, review adverse reactions that should be reported to his primary care provider.

Exercise

Explain the benefits of exercise, along with its purpose and effects on diabetes. Remember to warn your patient that hypoglycemia can occur with exercise. When you discuss exercise, you may want to review signs and symptoms of hypoglycemia and what to do if it occurs.

Diet

Review with your patient the diet prescribed by his primary care provider. Follow up on the teaching your patient received from his dietitian. A dietitian

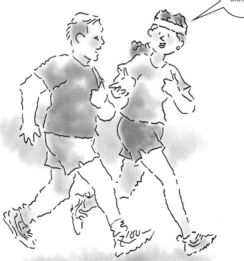

Check your blood glucose level before and after exercising to make sure your blood glucose level doesn't drop.

can effectively adjust a patient's diet to the patient's personal lifestyle. Your reinforcement of those instructions can greatly improve patient compliance.

Surgery

Your diabetic patient may benefit from transplantation of the pancreas or islet cells. Pancreas and islet cell transplants are being performed with increasing frequency on patients with severe, uncontrollable diabetes.

In addition to these new surgical procedures, current studies involving the immunosuppressant cyclosporine A suggest that the drug may eventually be used to combat islet cell–destroying antibodies in early type 1 diabetes.

If your patient is having surgery

For a patient having pancreas or islet cell transplant surgery, explain that he'll need to modify his insulin administration before, during, and after surgery. He'll need to review specific changes with his primary care provider and

Wait a minute! You mean I can be replaced?

will require more frequent monitoring to ensure adequate control of his blood glucose levels.

Teaching about self-monitoring

If your patient requires self-monitoring of his blood glucose levels, make sure he knows the acceptable range and what to do if he goes above or below it. He should also know how to properly clean and maintain his blood glucose monitor.

Tips for self-monitoring

Teach your patient these important points for self-monitoring his blood glucose levels:

• how to stick his finger to obtain the blood sample

• how to apply a droplet of blood to the test strip and how to read the results

• how proper technique and accurate timing help ensure reliable results

• why it is important to perform the test at the proper times

• if he experiences signs of hypoglycemia and hyperglycemia, why self-testing his blood glucose level is important to validate his symptoms.

Buying the right blood glucose monitor

To help the patient select the right monitor for him, advise that he ask these questions before purchasing one:

- Is cleaning and maintenance simple?
- What is the device's accuracy rating?
- Is the warranty reasonable?
- How much time is required to perform the test?
- How easy is the testing procedure?
- How much do test strips cost?
- What kind of technical support is provided?
- How extensive is the test memory?

To test your blood glucose level, you need just a few of us blood cells.

Monitoring hemoglobin A₁c

Your patient should know that his primary care provider will probably check his glycosylated hemoglobin (A_{1c}) level occasionally. Hemoglobin A_{1c} is a type of hemoglobin that results from glycosylation (glucose adherence to the hemoglobin protein) of normal hemoglobin A. The amount of glycosylation directly correlates with blood glucose levels.

Because hemoglobin A_{1c} accumulates over the 120-day life span of a red blood cell, measuring the hemoglobin A_{1c} level will show your patient's average blood glucose level over the previous 3 months or more.

Interpreting the hemoglobin A_{1c}

Ideally, your patient's hemoglobin A_{1c} should be no more than 1.5 times the normal level, which ranges from 3% to 6%. A high hemoglobin A_{1c} value with any blood glucose level suggests hyperglycemia over at least several weeks. A low value coupled with a high blood glu-

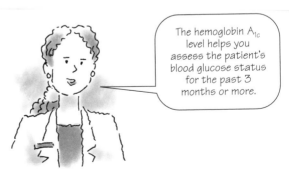

The hemoglobin A_{1c} level helps you assess the patient's blood glucose status for the past 3 months or more.

cose level suggests recent onset of hyperglycemia.

Long-term care concerns

Reassure your patient that he'll play a crucial role in preventing or minimizing diabetic complications by participating in his own care and recognizing and treating complications early, especially retinopathy, nephropathy, and neuropathy.

Explaining retinopathy

Tell your patient about the relationship between hypertension and retinopathy and about the steps he'll need to take to avoid or manage hypertension. Let him know that regular eye examinations are important — even when he doesn't have vision problems. Warn him that he must immediately report to his primary care provider episodes of blurred vision or visual halos.

Explaining nephropathy

Tell your patient that he'll need to avoid or manage hypertension that may occur as a result of nephropathy. Let him know that he should have his blood pressure checked frequently. Emphasize the importance of maintaining his ideal body weight, which will help keep his blood pressure under control. Finally, tell him to watch for urinary tract infections and to report signs or symptoms of infection to his primary care provider.

Meticulous skin care is crucial for preventing problems associated with peripheral vascular disease and neuropathy.

Explaining neuropathy

Tell the patient that the symptoms of this condition include altered sensation, burning, tingling, and numbness — all of which require immediate attention by his primary care provider. If your patient smokes, tell him that he should quit (or at least cut down). In addition, explain that he'll need to take meticulous care of his skin and feet. (See *Teaching about proper skin and foot care,* page 128.)

Illness and diabetes

Stress naturally occurs with the onset of an illness. This stress leads to the release of certain hormones that increase blood glucose levels. What's more, in many

(Text continues on page 131.)

Listen up!

Teaching about proper skin and foot care

Proper skin and foot care can help your patient avoid problems associated with peripheral vascular disease and neuropathy. To avoid even slight trauma, your patient should follow the guidelines described below.

Skin care

• Inspect the skin daily and look for small breaks, especially between the toes and around the toenails.
• Clean the skin with mild soap and warm water. Remind him to check water temperature first because neuropathy may prevent him from recognizing water that's too hot, thereby causing a burn. Bathwater should range between 90° and 95° F (32.2° to 35° C).
• Dry the skin gently to prevent tissue damage.
• Apply lotion after bathing to alleviate dry skin, but don't put lotion between the toes. Doing so can promote bacterial growth.

What to wear

• Wear clean cotton socks and underwear each day, and avoid tight-fitting garments that may impair leg and foot circulation.
• Wear leather shoes, if possible, because synthetic materials trap perspiration and may lead to fungal infections and blisters.
• Buy shoes late in the day, when the feet are swollen. Break in new shoes gradually to avoid blisters and subsequent infection.

Additional guidelines

• Never go barefoot, and always wear socks with shoes.
• Have a podiatrist remove corns and calluses.
• Cut toenails straight across, no shorter than the toe tip.
• Avoid using iodine or other harsh antiseptics on an injury.

Getting connected

Diabetes on the Internet

For more information on diabetes, check out these sources on the Internet.

American College of Foot and Angle Surgeons

www.acfas.org

This site provides descriptions of diabetic foot problems, causes, and ways to care for and prevent them. Check this site to obtain the latest information about foot care.

American Diabetes Association (ADA)

www.diabetes.org

This comprehensive site on diabetes contains general information about the disease, nutrition and exercise advice, recipes, news stories, and links to magazines and journals that cover diabetes. Current research, health insurance issues, and lists of doctors and education programs recognized by ADA are also included. Check this site first for information about diabetes.

American Dietetic Association

www.eatright.org

This site offers information about meal planning for people with diabetes. Check this site for the latest diet-related advice.

Diabetes Services Inc.

www.diabetesnet.com

This patient-friendly site is filled with information, including the way to figure insulin needs, a slide show on complications of diabetes, information on insulin pumps, tips and tricks for managing diabetes, research news, clinical trials, and topics specific to men and women. The site is appropriate for both patients and health care providers. Tell your patient about this site.

(continued)

Diabetes on the Internet *(continued)*

Joslin Diabetes Center

www.joslin.harvard.edu

This site offers an excellent beginner's guide to diabetes and is designed for the newly diagnosed patient and his family. Advise your patient to point his browser to this site for wide-ranging information about diabetes.

Mayo Health Clinic

www.mayohealth.org

This site contains the text of a comprehensive article on diabetes published in the renowned "Mayo Clinic Health Letter." Making effective use of graphics and links, the text presents complicated information clearly. This site is helpful for patients and health care providers.

National Diabetes Information Clearinghouse

www.niddk.nih.gov/health

This government-sponsored site provides information about diabetes for people with diabetes and their families as well as for health care providers. A secondary site provides information on neuropathy including an overview of this complication, its prevalence, its causes, its symptoms, the major types, its diagnosis and treatment, and the importance of good foot care. It also provides additional resources for patients with neuropathy and links to additional reading.

National Eye Institute

www.nei.nih.gov/publications

This site provides information on retinopathy for health care providers. You'll find definitions, reviews of symptoms, risk factors, prevention tips, detection information, and treatment guidelines. Photos illustrate what happens in the retinopathic eye. The site also provides a list of current research articles on retinopathy. Check this site for the latest information on eye-related damage secondary to diabetes. Note that the information offered on this site may be too complex for some patients.

Diabetes on the Internet (continued)
New York Online Access to Health (NOAH)
www.noah.cuny.edu
This site provides information about diabetes for patients in English and Spanish. It covers the basics of diabetes, its complications, care, and treatment and also provides links to other Web resources.

cases illness alters a person's food intake. For a nondiabetic patient, this change in dietary habit is insignificant. However, for a patient using insulin or taking an oral antidiabetic drug, the change can cause significant complications. Tell your patient to follow these guidelines when he becomes ill:

• Drink more fluids than usual.
• Monitor blood glucose levels more frequently than usual (about every 4 hours).
• If illness reduces dietary intake, spread half of his daily carbohydrate allowance over 24 hours.
• Immediately return to his prescribed diet after he feels better.
• Call his primary care provider if he can't eat or if he's vomiting; his insulin dose may need to be adjusted.
• Stock soft foods at home, such as custard, gelatin, and soft drinks, in case he's

unable to tolerate foods more difficult to digest.

Buddy up

Because hyperglycemia may worsen and lead to reduced awareness and perception, tell your patient not to stay alone when he's ill. For example, a family member or friend may need to contact a primary care provider if the patient is having trouble breathing or if he becomes sleepy or disoriented.

Documentation

Document all aspects of your teaching, and incorporate as many patient-teaching techniques as possible, including visual, auditory, and hands-on techniques. Complete documentation provides a legal record that not only shows what you've taught but also how the patient received the information and what aspects need to be clarified.

Quick quiz

1. Headache, diaphoresis, and palpitations are signs and symptoms of:
   A. hypoglycemia.
   B. hyperglycemia.
   C. DKA.

Answer: A. Headache, diaphoresis, faintness, palpitations, trembling, impaired vision, hunger, irritability, and personality changes are signs and symptoms of hypoglycemia.

2. Too little insulin, dietary noncompliance, or emotional distress may result in:
   A. hypoglycemia.
   B. hyperglycemia.
   C. insulin shock.

Answer: B. Too little insulin, dietary noncompliance, infection, illness, or emotional distress may result in hyperglycemia.

3. Current studies involving the immunosuppressant cyclosporine A suggest that the drug may eventually be used to:

    A. promote islet cell growth in type 2 diabetes.

    B. inhibit islet cell growth in early type 1 diabetes.

    C. combat islet cell–destroying antibodies in early type 1 diabetes.

Answer: C. Current studies involving the immunosuppressant cyclosporine A suggest that the drug may eventually be used to combat islet cell–destroying antibodies in early type 1 diabetes.

Scoring

✰✰✰ If you answered all three questions correctly, congratulations! You're our new Diabetes Teacher of the Year!

✰✰ If you answered two of three correctly, excellent! You're being awarded Insulin Instructor of the Month!

✰ If you answered fewer than two questions correctly, no problem. You're a shoo-in for the Up-and-Coming Diabetes Educator award!

Index

A

Acinar cells, 11i
Alpha cells, 11i, 17i, 19
Anaerobic exercise, 78. *See also* Exercise.
Appetite, increased, 55
Assessment, 53-68
    diagnostic tests in, 67-68
    focus for, 54
    for gestational diabetes, 68
    health history in, 54-56
    initial complaint in, 54-56
    past medical history in, 56
    physical examination in, 57-67. *See also* Physical examination.
    of previously diagnosed patients, 58
    socioeconomic history in, 56-57
Atherosclerosis
    pathophysiology of, 62-64
    prevention of, 40-41, 73-74

B

Beta cells, 11i
    defects of, 5
    destruction of, 5, 12i
    insulin production by, 19

C

Carbohydrates, 73t
    glycemic index for, 75, 76
Cardiac complications, prevention of, 49
Cardiovascular disease
    pathophysiology of, 62-64
    prevention of, 40-41, 73-74
Cell starvation, 22-27, 25t
Children and adolescents
    physical examination in, 66-67
    screening in, 33
Cholesterol, 37-38, 73-74
Clinical manifestations, 54-56
Coma, hyperosmolar, 27-28
    causes of, 103
    laboratory findings in, 99t-100t
    signs and symptoms of, 103
Complications, 97-111
    acute, 63t
    assessment for, 41-49
    cardiovascular, 40-41, 62-64, 73-74, 105
    chronic, 63t, 104-111, 126-132
    infectious, 44-45, 66
    of insulin therapy, 89-91
    nephropathy, 47-48, 64-65, 105-106, 126-127
    neuropathy, 48-49, 65-66, 107-109, 127
    of oral antidiabetic agents, 92-93

i refers to an illustration; t refers to a table.

i refers to an illustration; t refers to a table.

i refers to an illustration; t refers to a table.

i refers to an illustration; t refers to a table.

i refers to an illustration; t refers to a table.

i refers to an illustration; t refers to a table.

i refers to an illustration; t refers to a table.

i refers to an illustration; t refers to a table.

i refers to an illustration; t refers to a table.

Notes

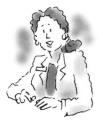

Notes

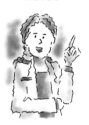